YELLOW FLAG

YELLOW FLAG

The
Civil War Journal
of Surgeon's Steward
C. Marion Dodson

EDITED BY

CHARLES ALBERT EARP

Charles Albert Earp

MHS
Maryland Historical Society
Baltimore

$\mathcal{M}_{d}\mathcal{H}_{s}$

The Maryland Historical Society
extends special thanks to the
Joseph Meyerhoff Family Charitable Funds
for generous support of this publication.

Library of Congress Cataloging-in-Publication Data
Dodson, C. Marion.
   Yellow flag : the Civil War journal of surgeon's steward, C. Marion
Dodson / edited by Charles Albert Earp.
      p. cm.
   Includes bibliographical references and index.
   ISBN 0-938420-79-8 (pbk. : alk. paper)
   1. Dodson, C. Marion—Diaries. 2. Physicians' assistants—United
States—Diaries. 3. United States. Navy—Biography. 4. United
States—History—Civil War, 1861–1865—Personal narratives. 5.
United States—History—Civil War, 1861–1865—Medical care.
6. Yellow fever—Louisiana—New Orleans—History—19th
century. 7. United States—History—Civil War, 1861–1865—
Blockades. 8. Saint Michaels (Md.)—Biography. I. Earp, Charles
Albert. II. Title.

E621 .D63 2002
973.7'75–dc21
                                                              2001055832

Printed in the United States of America.
The paper used in this publication meets the minimum
requirements of the American National Standard for Information
Sciences Permanence of Paper for Printed Library Materials
ANSI Z39.48-1984

CONTENTS

ACKNOWLEDGMENTS   VII
LIST OF ILLUSTRATIONS   IX
INTRODUCTION   XI

1. U.S.S. POCAHONTAS
Philadelphia to New Orleans
March 1, 1864 – June 3, 1864
West Gulf Blockading Squadron
June 4, 1864 – October 7, 1864
1

2. U.S.S. ARKANSAS
Yellow Fever
October 8, 1864 – November 2, 1864
69

3. U.S.S. HOLLYHOCK
Destruction of the C.S.S. *William H. Webb*
November 3, 1864 – April 30, 1865
89

4. U.S.S. BERMUDA
New Orleans to Philadealphia
May 1, 1865 – June 1, 1865
Maryland
June 5, 1865 – November 22, 1929
133

ADDENDA   145
BIBLIOGRAPHY   149
INDEX   151

ACKNOWLEDGMENTS

I am indebted to many people for assistance in the preparation of this book, including: the staffs of the Maryland Historical Society, the Nimitz Library at the United States Naval Academy, the Naval Research Center and National Archives, and the Mariner's Museum. Terry Reimer of the National Museum of Civil War Medicine provided essential clarification of medical terminology. Dr. William Reichel and Pharmacist Amy Bittner also contributed to this phase of the research. Don Juedes of the Milton S. Eisenhower Library of the Johns Hopkins University helped with computer searches for source documents and images. Daniel Carroll Toomey permitted use of the Dodson image from the original in his collection. Dr. Robert I. Cottom, Publications Director at the Maryland Historical Society, was a constant source of encouragement and technical support. My sincere thanks go to all of them.

LIST OF ILLUSTRATIONS

The Dodson house in St. Michaels, Maryland, n.d.   2

Robert Dodson   4

Camp Carroll, Baltimore, Md.   4

Baltimore Harbor, 1863   5

Philadelphia Navy Yard   8

Union volunteers welcomed in Philadelphia   11

U.S.S. *Pocahontas* at sea   22

Map of the Gulf of Mexico   42–43

Pages from Dodson's hymnal   56–57

Levee at New Orleans   88

U.S.S. *Hollyhock*   103

Map of the Mississippi Delta   118

U.S.S. *Richmond*   123

Lieutenant Charles Reed   125

C.S.S. *William H. Webb* after being run aground
and set afire   127

Philadelphia Navy Yard   130

Dodson's house in St. Michaels, circa 1895   136

C. Marion Dodson   138

Dodson's certficate of membership in the
Grand Army of the Republic   138

INTRODUCTION

In the manuscript collection of the Maryland Historical Society in Baltimore is the Civil War journal of Dr. C. Marion Dodson who served as a surgeon's steward in the Union Navy. Apparently a druggist in civilian life, his naval duties were often more akin to those of a present-day paramedic or physician's assistant. The journal is more than two hundred pages long, is perfectly preserved and, with few exceptions, completely legible. He wrote well and was a keen observer of people and events.

The journal covers the period from March 1864 to June 1865 during his service on three different ships. A native of St. Michaels, Maryland, Dodson enlisted in Philadelphia, where he joined the crew of the U.S.S. *Pocahontas,* which was undergoing repairs. The first section of the journal recounts his enlistment, shipboard duties fitting out the ship's pharmacy, and his social life ashore. When the *Pocahontas* finally sailed, he wrote about the long voyage from Philadelphia to her duty station in the West Gulf blockading squadron, enlivening the account of the voyage with descriptions of shipboard routine, the personalities of his shipmates, and sights seen along the way.

From May to October, 1864, the *Pocahontas* was stationed off the coast of Texas. Dodson's account of blockade duty is climaxed by his account of the death and burial at sea of Dr. Mann, his superior officer and good friend.

During the month of October, one of the most dramatic periods of his service occurred when he volunteered to serve aboard the U.S.S. *Arkansas,* the site of a yellow fever epidemic. Dodson, then only twenty-two years old, arrived on board to discover that the ship's surgeon was down with the disease. When the *Arkansas* was finally released from quarantine Dodson was reassigned.

His next duty was aboard the U.S.S. *Hollyhock*, a combination dispatch, tug, and fire boat based in New Orleans, where he had charge of the medical department. The journal records his observations on duties aboard this vessel and his surprisingly active social life in the city. The high point of this section is Dodson's vivid description of the *Hollyhock's* battle with the Confederate ram *William H. Webb*, which resulted in the destruction of that vessel.

Dodson was discharged May 13, 1865, returned to Philadelphia on the U.S.S. *Bermuda*, then made his way to Baltimore and finally home via the same bay steamer on which he had left fifteen months before.

In an addenda in the journal Dodson described the ships with which he was associated and set forth a detailed and graphic description of the symptoms and progression to death of yellow fever. With the journal at the Maryland Historical Society is a photograph of the U.S.S. *Hollyhock* and a copy of a music score in Dodson's handwriting that he prepared as choir director aboard the *Pocahontas*. Copies accompany the transcript along with a postwar photograph of Dr. Dodson as a member of the Maryland Naval Veterans Association.

After the war he became a physician and practiced medicine in Baltimore for many years. His death at his country home in St. Michaels at the age of eighty-seven is poignantly described in his obituary.

CHARLES ALBERT EARP
TIMONIUM, MARYLAND
JULY 2001

The yellow flag
was hoisted on Civil War
naval ships to indicate that an
epidemic of yellow fever had struck,
and that the ship was under quarantine.
At the time, yellow fever
was an often fatal disease
of unknown origin,
for which there was no cure.

I.

U.S.S. POCAHONTAS

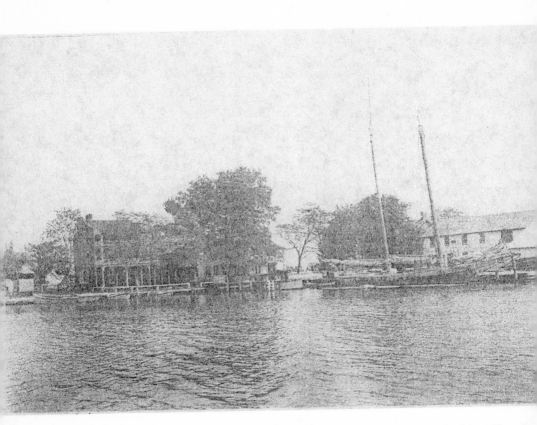

The Dodson house in St. Michaels, Maryland, n.d. (Chesapeake Bay Maritime Museum.

Philadelphia to New Orleans
MARCH 1, 1864 – JUNE 3, 1864

March 1, 1864

On Steamer *Champion*.[1] In company of mother came to Baltimore (envoule for Philadelphia) Called to see Brother Rich who was clerking at the Fountain Hotel. From that point we went to his house up East Pratt street. A few hours at that place Bro Rob[2] came in [illegible]. He was with his regiment encamped at Camp Carroll Western Section of the city. Rob proposed a visit to Miss Applegarths on High St. We spent a very pleasant evening. I found quite a number of gentlemen there and I soon learned it

1. The *Champion* was one of the many Chesapeake Bay steamers which, with the railroad, were the principal means of transportation throughout central Maryland and to Maryland's Eastern Shore. Such service continued well into the twentieth century, and the editor remembers making the round trip from Baltimore to Norfolk shortly before the service was discontinued. See David C. Holly, *Chesapeake Steamboats: Vanished Fleet* (Centreville, Md.: Tidewater Publishers, 1994) for an account of this bygone period.

2. The Dodsons have been a prominent family in St. Michaels, Talbot County, Maryland for many years. Captain William Dodson commanded an artillery company in the War of 1812 when the British attacked St. Michaels. Dodsons also served as postmaster and newspaper editor, and several captained luxuriously furnished packets providing passenger service between St. Michaels and Baltimore. See Oswald Tilghman, *History of Talbot County, Maryland 1661–1861*, 2 vols. (Baltimore: Clearfield Company, 1997), 1:317–18, 2:31, 395–96, 404.

Richard S. Dodson is listed as a bookkeeper at the Maltby House in the *Baltimore City Directory, 1860*. He apparently changed jobs. Robert Dodson was Assistant Surgeon in the 1st Maryland Cavalry, U.S. Volunteers. See *History and Roster of Maryland Volunteers in the War of 1861–1865*, 2 vols. (Baltimore: Press of Guggenheimer, Weil & Co., 1898–99), volume 1.

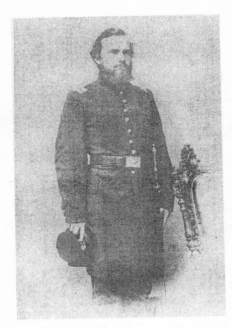

Robert Dodson, brother of C. Marion Dodson, in uniform. (Chesapeake Bay Maritime Museum.) His regiment, the 1st Maryland Cavalry, was encamped at Camp Carroll (below) when Dodson first arrived in Baltimore. (Maryland Historical Society.)

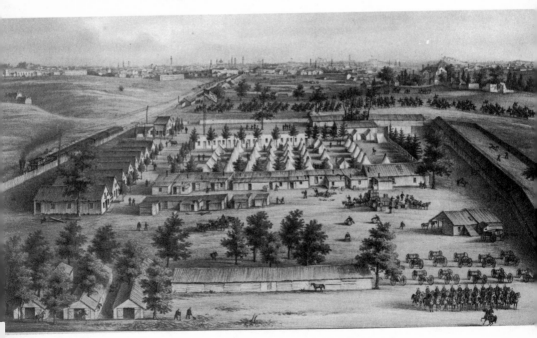

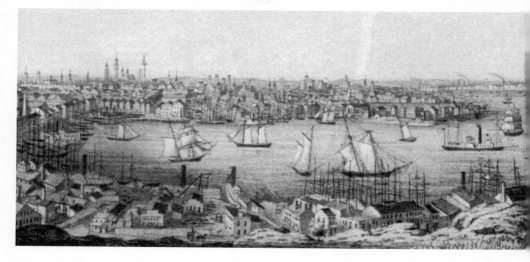

View of Baltimore Harbor in 1863. (Maryland Historical Society.)

was quite popular to denounce the vigor of government in checking the Rebellion for there seems to be a loud cry against the actions she is putting forth at this time

March 2, 3, 4

Spent some days in Baltimore. Occasional visits to Camp Carroll with Brother Rob I find they are seemingly enjoying their sins. One day Dr secured the major's horse for me and we enjoyed a ride. Extended mine to Mr Phelps on the Philadelphia Road. During these days mother was not with us stopping at Maria's and I had quite a pleasant time. She is quite free from any domestic cares. to pass her time very easily she would occasionally make a trip to see some of her old friends during the day but in the evenings we were gathered together and had a social chat. I told her last night that I was going to consomate my plan that I had named to her before we left Talbot [Co] to join the Navy. She says whatever I think best to act upon. She did not chose to give a full amen.

March 5th 1864

Took the morning train[3] to Philadelphia. The day was exceedingly close and damp. Added to this the train was full of passengers and some how or other there was not enough room, many having to stand until camp stools were brought. We had too much [————] company as far as Marcus Hook (I think that is the name of the station) but at that place some started to leave the cars and gave us a little better breathing and seating capacity. Came to Philadelphia 3 PM. Called to see George Benson Thos Willey Chas Benson from Saint Michaels who had been living here for some time. Found them in good boarding house so took up my quarters there also.

March 6th

A damp and rainy day taking a good rest at the boarding house. In the afternoon feeling a little refreshed called to see Misses MHH.[4] They seemed surprised to see me. After a little while we went to call on Miss ADH. Being Sunday went to church in the afternoon. Spent evening at Mr Love's. I found in this family truly a Christian atmosphere and much reminding me of those whom I had left at home. Later in the evening called to see Mr Loders. The same Christian home presented itself for instead of the [————] and light conversation one generally finds prominent in most City homes the Solemnity of the day and its duties are observed and I left that place fully impressed with the thought that even in confusion of a bustling city there are spots quite [————] and beautified by a constant communion with a kind and loving "Father."

3. The trip was via the Philadelphia, Wilmington and Baltimore railroad.

4. Dodson seems to have had numerous acquaintances in Philadelphia who cannot now be identified. He was always very discrete in his references to the fairer sex and rarely reveals the name of a woman friend. In his entry for March 8, 1864, however, he does identify "Miss ADH" as Anne D. Hahn.

March 7th 1864

This morning feeling fully rested and having in mind the principal cause of my visit to Philadelphia started for the Navy Yard. I had heard of the many vessels that were being fitted out from that place and thought perhaps some one of them would offer some position that I could fill. When arrived at the Yard found several steamers, iron clads, etc being "fitted out" as they term it. One vessel seemed to please my fancy. She seemed "neat and trim." A brig rigged, screw propellor. There was a large force of workmen, painters, riggers, machinists, etc and though from a distance the *Pocahontas*[5] looked well, on board a perfect Babel was there. Seeing men going to and fro I thought I would take a peep myself. I am told she will not go into Commission so visitors can have access.

All of her officers are ordered although only a few are on board. They are boarding on shore till the painters are through. After looking around a young man comes up to me and says in a friendly way "What do you think of the "Po-ka-hon-tas" accompanying the speech with a sort of smile which I shall never forget. He belongs to the Engineering Department of the steamer he said He [————] Rodney Carter is his name and said

---

5. The USS *Pocahontas* was a 694-ton, screw steamer, rated as a second class sloop and armed with six guns. She was originally purchased by the navy as the *City of Boston* in 1855 at a cost of $57,000. She was fitted out at Norfolk on March 30, 1861, for the relief of Fort Sumter and was present at the surrender of the Federal garrison. She subsequently served on the Potomac River, along the Atlantic coast and in the Gulf of Mexico. Ordered back to Philadelphia , she was severely damaged in a storm during which her smokestack blew over. She was in the Philadelphia Navy Yard for repairs when Dodson first saw her. The *Pocahontas* was decommissioned by the navy in late 1868. *Dictionary of American Naval Fighting Ships,* 8 vols. (Washington, D.C.: U.S. Department of the Navy, Office of the Chief of Naval Operations, 1991), 5:332–33; *Official Records of the Union and Confederate Navies in the War of the Rebellion,* 30 vols. (Washington, D.C.: Government Printing Office, 1894), Series I, Vols. 4, 12, 20–22 passim. Hereafter cited as *OR*.

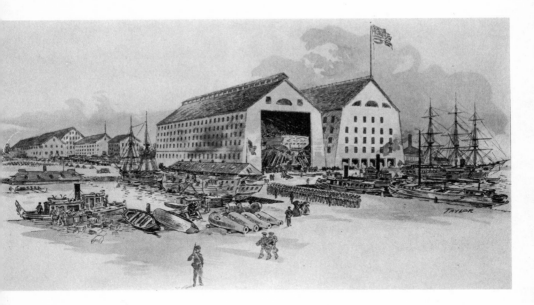

Philadelphia Navy Yard. (From Frank H. Taylor, Philadelphia in the Civil War, 1861–1865 *{Philadelphia: By the City, 1913}.)*

"he has been to sea before." In spite of the torn up condition of the ship I certainly like her appearance.

When I started out to join the Navy I knew nothing of one's requirements or what was expected. I was told on every ship there was a miniature drug store and a druggist was appointed to it whose duty was just as on land to prepare and compound medicines. Strange to say I found this position vacant. Mr. Carter as soon as I told him I was a druggest insisted that I immediately see Dr. Mann,[6] and make application as there were many after it.

6. Rodney F. Carter, Acting 3d Assistant Engineer, and Dr. George R. Mann, Acting Assistant Surgeon, the two men first mentioned on this date, would become his closest friends. Dr. Mann, appointed September 21, 1861, is mentioned a number of times during fleet operations in the North Carolina sounds and commanded an assault column during the unsuccessful attack on Fort Sumter in 1863. In the navy, "Acting" meant temporary and was applied to all volunteers who were not members of the regular navy. Edward W. Callahan, ed., *List of Officers of the United States Navy and of the*

The doctor being quite particular had deferred his choice til all applicants had stood examination. Later in the day called to see Dr. Mann, asked particulars in regard to duties, etc. At his suggestion made application for the position. Offered wine, asked to come into the parlor and to stand examination, prefacing it by saying his "answer would be given in a day or so" before the steamer would go into commission.

While in the parlor as one would suppose he asked many questions and I thought Dr. Mann would have done credit to have been a regular board of examiners. After he seemed to tire of medicine and druggist duties he retired for a few minutes, bringing papers etc in. In the interim wine had been offered. Dr. Says "after a little reflection, I have changed my plans and here is your application. It will only need the approval of the commanding officer so you report to him at the Continental Hotel for approval on the morrow and at some future time I will tell you why I was so soon in making up my mind." T'was quite late in the evening when I returned to my friends who had thought me bound homeward before this. I did not say anything to them of my adventure but went to bed with my head full of thoughts of "life on the ocean wave."

March 8th

Early in the morning called to see Dr. Mann. We went to the Continental hotel and received the approval of my appointment. Dr says as several days will be before the ship is ready I had better take a grant of absence. In the evening went up to see Miss Ann D Hahn.[7] During the conversation a trip with the

---

Marine Corps from 1775 to 1900 (New York: Haskell House, 1969), gives a brief biography of each man but does not cite the ships on which they served. Lewis Randolph Hamersly, ed., *A Naval Encyclopedia* (Philadelphia, 1881), 18.

7. Dodson was apparently quite friendly with the Hahn family in

Perkiomen was debated and finally approved of so we said good
bye to meet equiped for the trip to "Sunderland College" on the
morrow. The ladies it seemed had pleasant memories centered
around the college. One had a father living close and had spent
much of her school days within its walls. The other had a sister
at this time attending the same place. And I hardly need add I
had a special desire to see how the sister was coming on, previously having spent a few days in her company in Washington.

March 9th

I had hardly supposed yesterday when my thoughts had been
where "green vissaged var" that they would have been so soon
"smoothed" by the pleasant company and bright prospects of a
trip to the college but all this was realized when we found
ourselves pleasantly on the broad veranda of Sunderland's School.
Our trip had all the variety one generally experiences when a
stage coach ride terminates. The journey on cars far as
Norristown. Then the jolting. I fully agree with the one who says
"good place to judge complexion of disposition is the ride in a
stage." Went to a little hotel close and took supper. In evening
called to see the sister of Miss AD. The ground around the
building is much improved presenting a cheerful and inviting
appearance.

March 10th

According to agreement last evening went over to the school
and, in company of Washington friend we further viewed the
professor's grounds but as they did not seem to be the prominent attraction will pass them over without further notice.

Philadelphia, who are often mentioned during his stay there. One suspects
his principal interest in the Hahns is Miss Anne.
    I was unable to determine the meaning of "perkioman" referred to on this
date. Perhaps it is the name of some mode of transportation of the time.

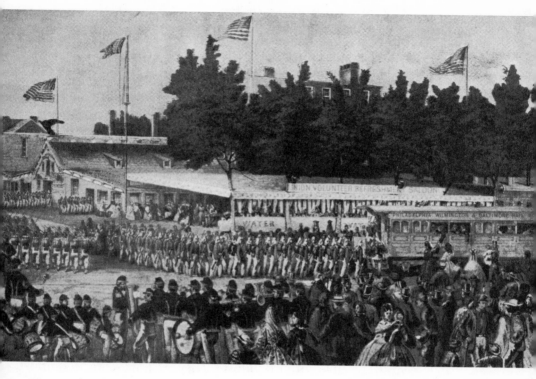

Union volunteers moving south received a warm welcome in Philadelphia, where citizens provided banquets for entire regiments. Dodson probably witnessed such a scene during his stay there. (From Frank H. Taylor, Philadelphia in the Civil War, 1861–1865 *{Philadelphia: by the City, 1913}.)*

Something seemed to make the time pass pleasantly for in a short time I heard someone call out "stage for Norristown will soon be here." Thought of that stage and what amount of fortitude necessary to endure its jerks could not be long debated. So, saying a hearty adieu we start, arriving at Philadelphia in time enough to visit the store where the young men are employed who left St. Michaels last year. Thomas Willey is in a book store Benson & Bro in shoe stores.

March 11th

Today most of the time at the boarding house with the Maryland boys. While there Edward Brownell from St. Michaels came in. He seemed quite nervous. He had been drafted in Talbot Co and had left the section. He thought perhaps I would inform on him but he can have no fear from that source. I shall never speak of it. Later in the evening called to see some ladies. One charmed me with song that reminds me of the pleasures of my home life. One, even so short a time away and loves home as I, cant help having a few sad thoughts and suppose they are one of the necessary bequests to make one give it its fullest appreciation.

March 12th 1864

Reported to Dr Mann aboard the *Pocahontas.* He asks me, before taking my duties upon myself, to assist him in getting his papers in shape and then I can have time to arrange the Dispensary or drug store to my fancy.

Today the noise of the boiler making is fearful, everyplace seems to be alive with machinists. They are putting forth quite an effort to have ship ready for sea.

Then there are a lot of painters. What a smell of [———] paints, oil, etc. Brother Clay's paint room is a perfumed place. Carpenters and joiners join in the train and make things lively, I find, working for the government. A man who lifts a 12 foot board does a big thing but when he calls 3 or 4 others and then all assist to place it on wheels he does a bigger one.

13th

Yesterday drew $50 from the Navy Agent. Today am on board. The carpenters are fitting up little rooms with berths, tables, etc. The room I am to have for the Dispensary is painted though hardly dry. A counter is in, prescription scales in case & a somewhat of an "outfit" stored away in closets under counter etc and printed list of stock on hand points to a small allowance to what the schedule entitles us. So in the morning I will call the doctor's attention to it. In the meanwhile a carpenter is turned over to me to do all that is necessary. Very little shelving is required as each [———] bottle is in an iron clamp which screws up to the wall or partition which being regular gives a good appearance and will not tumble over should the steamer roll. Glad to escape the smells and noise of the day I went to the boarding house.

14th

On board most of the day. Called Dr Mann's attention to the small portion of medical stores. Dr. says smiling "You have a form among your papers that tells exactly what is allowed on board this steamer and when I order a thing shall expect to find it." I remembered that remark and when I ordered stock you would have observed that there were very few omissions. During the afternoon I went to see some of the iron clads (monitors) and what huge structures. Seemed their excessive height would totally unfit them to be of any service. Hardly able to float and run if they swim at all. Would be like an iron pot. One of these boats, the *Towanda*,[8] was a curiosity.

15th of March

Spent most time on the *Pocahontas*.

March 16, 1864

Pocahontas is ready for sea. Went into commission hauled out from the wharf and dropped anchor off Navy Yard. My stock of drugs, chemicals, instruments, etc came. The best portion of the morning spent arranging bottles, opening goods, etc. A temporary nurse is detailed and turned over to me who is to do duties in the sick bay

8. USS *Towanda* was a 536-ton, twin screw, double turreted monitor armed with eighteen guns. *OR*:II:1, *Statistical Data of US Ships*, 225.

department. There are no sick for him to attend to so I found one
for him. Received from the Receiving Ship a portion of a crew.
Seamen are quite scarce. The *"Powhatan"*[9] is ahead of us and took
all who could. She is a beautiful boat and expect to hear of good
reports when she turns up.

March 17

Off Philadelphia Navy Yard. It is very cold and frequent snow
storms are upon us. During the day several men came on board as
part crew. Quite a poor excuse for "bone and muscle" except one
large man. He was a good specimen. He was the captain of a
blockade runner. It seems with the others he was taken and they
gave him choice of prison or shipping in the Navy. He chose the
latter. He is to be named as boatswains mate on board and as far
as he looks will perform his duties well. As I look at him I think
how much out of position he seems. He is the best looking man
on board and if he had been in good uniform would have been a
credit to the appearance of a full grown admiral when on the
Quarter deck.

18 off Philadelphia

Weather continues very cold. Stormy winds and snowing. The
Delaware so rough that it with the greatest effort the crew of
the cutter can go on shore so little communication is kept up
with the shore. Last night I could not get warm enough though
good blankets. I thought this was something like the crews of
the different Polar expeditions trying to find a warm corner. Such
a spell is telling upon health of the men forward. Found several
unfit for duty cough and cold order of the day.

One fellow found necessary to blister, a genuine "Son of Erin."
He shipped as "ordinary seaman." His fittness may be judged

9. USS *Powhatan* was a 2,415-ton, side-wheel, wood steamer, rated a first
class sloop, number of guns varied over time. *OR*:II:1:183.

14

when he stated he had never slept in a hammock before or as he expressed his indignation for the Navy. Says "I'm a gentleman you know and always slept in a bed but here they hang me up in a baggy hammock. No wonder I am hacking and coughing bad luck to the man who paid me a bounty."

19 Still the bay of Philadelphia

Cool and dull day. Dr Mann went to New York only a few of the officers are on board and things are quite cheerless. I shall soon turn in and see if some sleep will make time pass. Every place on the spar deck is damp and you would smile to see who come as seaman drawn up and pretty much used up. Such sailors, a little blast seems to unfit them for farther use. Frequent applications to go on sick list. Well some of them I'm sorry for, particularly the landsmen. Some are from comfortable homes in Philadelphia. Their duties are quite a task scrubbing of decks, polishing bright work rowing the cutters, etc.

March 20th

Spent short time on shore. Called at a drug store corner of 4th and Noble. Made arrangements if my trunk came to have forwarded. In the evening returned to the *Pocahontas*. It is a dull and dreary place. No bright glow of coal fire or glare of gas light to make things genial and comfortable. No warmth no light only a few lanterns throw out a melancholy light. I am alone in my Dispensary at repose if one could so interpret it. Under the most favorable circumstances with friends such a scene could hardly be endured. Well here I am how! why! My duties and position have not been once thought upon. I shall wait 'till a more cheering state of things exist before contemplating what is before me.

March 21

A message from home. Charlie Blades came from *St. Michaels*. I had written to him and before knowing the full duties of nurse had suggested that he accept that position but by the time of his arrival I had seen there were many pleasanter positions for him and suggested that for a day or so he would try for something better. So he soon received a good place on board the *USS Massachusetts.* I was much pleased with this though could Charlie have gotten a good place on the *Pocahontas* I would have been glad of his company. Charlie brought on my trunk which added much to my comfort by its contents such as a careful mother would plan and I soon saw many things that brought to mind Home bed cloths etc. All had been there before and tonight if a few tears are on my pillow the cause is known.

March 22

When Charlie left the ship I thought I would go up and see him. He had taken quarters at same boarding house where the Maryland boys were. When I awoke found we had quite a storm upon us; in fact it blew so hard as to prevent any communication with the shore. No cutter left the boat that day. We were certainly having "blue days." We have a very good table though not much heart to eat. Our surroundings are not very cheering. We debated at dinner as to our future mode of living. What article of use who would be caterer of the mess and what stock of provisions would be required. All in our company are inexperienced and any suggestion from a *"knowing one"* we put it down. As few days are supposed to be in port we should soon shape up matters.

March 23rd

"The sun at last shines." Yes we have once more seen the sun a welcome visitor bringing cheer to all of us. Such drying of cloths, getting up things in general. Sailors unfolding sails; if there were ever a time when hearts and bodies needed cheer and sunshine tis now and today promises to do the thing. I was favored by a visit

from some ladies, the Mss H,[10] and not knowing exactly naval
Etiquit was grossly neglectful and passed them their dinner or
failed to ask them for as I subsequently learned they would have
taken dinner but we failed to ask them as all things had been
cleared away. Well I think they did not feel much ignored for
they know how unsettled things were on the steamer.

24

The day is cold though not any rain till night. We are yet
debating around the table the best man to take charge of affairs
in the eating department and now a *knowing one*[11] speaks up.
"We did so and so on the *Ship Marion*." All eyes are on the
speaker a tall lean & lank: true specimen *Yankee*. What, have you
been to sea? An afirmative answer and that settles the matter.
Before we adjourn each has handed him $18 to get our "lay in"
as he terms it. Our crockery, provisions, etc. As there were seven
of us our lank friend [had] a good bank capital to commence
operations and we had fresh provisions while in port but have to
provide for our future when at sea. Hence the need of a caterer.

25th

Found a storm raging. The ship is dragging anchor as a preventive steam is ordered. This adds much to our comfort as it makes
it quite warm in the berth deck and as my quarters are between
the boilers and large range where the cooking is done I am
pleasantly situated even if it does make me think what will be
the condition of things when down south in summer. "Sufficient

10. Probably the Hahn sisters mentioned earlier.

11. The "knowing one" was Augustus Barnes, the Paymaster's Clerk,
who appears frequently throughout the journal in a good-natured way as a
sort of comic relief. Dodson obviously liked him. He appears on a list of
officers of the USS *Pocahontas*, April 1, 1864, in List of Officers on Vessels,
Volume II, bound manuscripts, Record Group 45, National Archives.
Hereafter cited as Officers List ms.

for the day is the evil" and I accept the comfort with a good grace.

Have several cases of Bronchitis on board. Dr. Mann is absent and found that constantly expecting him I have blistered some and freely wrapping [them] up in close garments and do as much as circumstances will permit.[12]

26th Philadelphia Navy Yard

After going around sick call and making them as comfortable as possible gaining the deck the officer on watch says "don't you want to go on shore." A cutter is called and will leave in a few minutes. I went had leave til 6 PM. As doctor was absent I had to be on board at night. Called to see the ladies at Dr. H. Found the sister from Sunderland's school there and had a very pleasant time with them. Upon my return to the wharf found the storm brewing so severe no boat came off so had to spend the night on shore. Went to some sort of a German hotel close to the Navy Yard. When I went to bed found no bed cloths. Called up porter who smilingly said "there your quarters." It appears they use a feather bed for covering. When once in one sleeps very nicely.

27 Sunday

First divine service chaplain from the receiving ship *Princeton* came on board

28

Still regular March blows. Spent most of the day in my Dispensary reading. In fact did not go upon the gun deck this day.

12. "Blisters" refers to the application of spanish fly (*Ceratum Cantharidis*) or some other substance used as an irritant to cause counter-irritation of the skin, which was believed to aid in healing. To treat bronchitis the blistering ointment was probably applied to the chest. In "wrapping [bronchitis patients] up in close garments," Dodson means tight clothing or a dressing to cover the ointment.

Found the heat from the boilers made an agreeable change in the temperature

29

Some bronchitis Pneumonia. Quite a large sick report. Dr still absent and found much of the day devoted to medicines for the sick and in the extreme bows of the ship I have formed a sick bay and installed Randall my nurse who has charge of affairs. We have several cots in place and the sick are placed in them and made as comfortable as possible. There are three men who if I can prevail upon our Captain will send to the hospital tomorrow.

March 30th

Dr being absent I saw Captain Jones[13] and explained the case of the three men that I wanted removed. So soon as he gave his permission went to the hospital with them and after a little "red tape" business it was soon over, balance of the day spent in the city. In the evening called to the Dr. Saw Miss W.

March 31st

Find quite a stormy day upon us. Dr seems to have taken quite a trip, nothing heard from him. Some say "We are to sail in a day or so." Things dont seem to point out that way to me. Even the few seamen we had have been taken from us and sent to other vessels to fix up complement having the first turn. Not much of interest going on on board.

13. The captain of the *Pocahontas* at the time Dodson joined her was Meriwether P. Jones, a graduate of the Naval Academy who had attained the rank of lieutenant commander on July 16, 1862 (Callahan, *List of Officers*). He died on April 11, 1866. Often the rank cited by Dodson is higher than the officers' official rating. Rank varied with the size of the vessel on which an officer was then serving.

The evening visit was to the Hahns and Miss W. may have been his Washington friend previously mentioned.

April 1st 1864

Off Philadelphia Navy Yard. Seems that we are not making much progress toward sailing. Of course I am not in a position to know much of our future but for myself I am getting quite tired of such life and wish we were off. Left the ship in the morning called to see Frank Hahn who insisted that I take supper and spend the evening with him. Did so meeting his sisters. Soon Miss M.A.N.[14] came in. Also met a Cuban MD who seemed to be quite agreeable though he had an opinion of how the war should be conducted and of course did not accord with the doings of the government. Later in the evening returned to the Pocahontas.

April 2

No indication of sailing. At night there was somewhat of a stir on board. A small boat was seen approaching was hailed by a mate reported to the engineer who also hailed it but by a skillful and preconcerted plan it swung around our bows and succeeded in carrying off one of our sailors

April 3

April showers. We have a little of the rough element in our crew. Some had gutter whiskey and behaved very badly. Two men are so violent and troublesome that they were placed in irons and carried below where they are to spend the night "drunken fools." A little liberty on shore they could not stand it and have forfeited the respect of all by their beastly conduct.

4 April on board

I am going to send two more men to the hospital and will go on shore myself. Am to pay a visit to the steamer *Bermuda*[15] to day if

14. Could not be identified.
15. USS *Bermuda* was an unarmed, 1,238-ton screw steamer used as a

I can find time. Find this an iron steamer captured from the blockade runners. I found a young man on board same occupation he had posted me on many points as to duty, position etc all of which I found came in good time.

April 5

Dr Mann came assisted in different department dealing out drugs then planned a change in the sleeping department of the sick. Dr found several men unfit for duty.

April 6th

Went on shore took a sick man to the hospital in company of one of the officers enjoyed a little stroll through the city.

April 7

Day sun is quite hot. Several sailors come on board. All pass examination except one. Am feeling badly today. Yesterday exposed myself too much to the sun.

April 8th On board USS Pocahontas

Wrote several letters home. Mr Boggs and Carlton[16] master mates were transferred to the *Ticonderoga* and sailed for China. They appear to be fine specimins of officers and we all regret their leaving us.

From the 8th to the 12th Off Philadelphia

Some of the evenings I would ride up to Dr. H and one trip from there was favored by a walk with Miss N who came as far as the

---

supply ship. She formerly had been a blockade runner until captured by the USS *Mercedita* in 1862 and purchased from the Navy Prize Court. See OR:II:1:45. Dodson returned to Philadelphia on this ship after his discharge from the navy.

16. Probably Mate Archibald G. Boggs and Acting Ensign Thomas I. Carleton. Callahan, *List of Officers*.

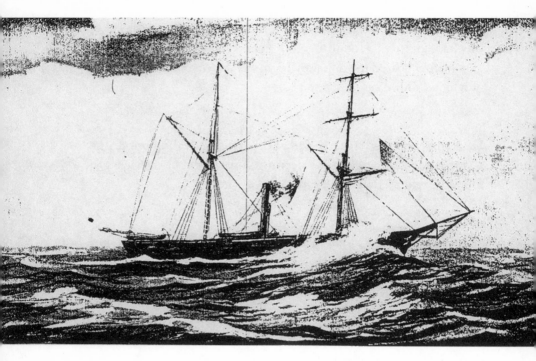

U.S.S. Pocahontas *at sea. (Naval History Center, Washington, D.C.)*

Navy Yard (this was the last evening before we sailed) being quite a pleasant one. We enjoyed the long walk and when I had seen her safely on the cars for her return went on board the *Pocahontas.*

April 14th 1864

At last the ship is ready all hands on board steam up and we are soon gliding down the Delaware. Made New Castle. Spent the night off this place.

April 15

Sun in the morning. Quit New Castle after a pleasant sail down the bay came to Cape Henlopen and anchored.

16 off Cape Henlopen

During the night a severe case of "Delerium Tremans" occurred.[17] Man trying to jump overboard. Dr ordered strong
opiates. Managed to keep him quiet a little. In the morning a
cutter was lowered and he was sent to the USS *Saratoga* lying
close to the "break water." I went over in the boat and gave the
necessary papers. An ensign was in charge of the cutter. We soon
had the man over the *Saratoga's* sides. As to his final doom the
noise he made we care very little.

April 17th

On the Atlantic. Since ship rolling many seasick. Our Captain
read morning service[18] on quarter deck and as many as could
stand gave him their presence. At supper only a very few wanted
anything. Even our *knowing one* who "had been there before" was
absent and his long form could be seen stretched out in his berth
from which an occasional groan told that all was not going well
with him. There were many scenes and incidents occuring on
this first day on the ocean that was amusing. I must say as long as
I kept on Deck and took in pure air in abundance all went well
but as soon as I went to my room everything seemed to be upside
down. Glad to rest. Went to bed leaving the ship according to
officers calculations off Cape Charles Va.

April 18

On the ocean Health of men good The bright sun to-day makes

17. Delirium tremens, a severe, sometimes fatal form of delirium due to
alcoholic withdrawal following a period of sustained intoxication. It is also
symptomatic of opium addiction. "Strong opiates" probably refers to
morphine, which would have a definite effect on DTs.

18. Dodson was a religious young man and directed the ship's choir at
worship services. He mentions this role frequently in the journal. Among
his papers is a hymn book in his handwriting. He apparently had some
musical training.

things quite cheerful. I have found a very pleasant place to pass time away. Upon the fore top the cross trees are floored over except spaces enough for the men to crawl through. This makes a platform about 6 + 6 feet. Mr Cromburger Captain's clerk[19] came up. Also Dr Mann. We spent most of the day thus. While up there I have a good time for contemplation. My comrades are quite drowsy and occasionally raise themselves up to see if any unusual sights are to be witnessed but nothing can be decerned except the vast expanse of water. We can lay down and have plenty of room here so we can often take naps here as netting will protect us from falling. Dr calls the messenger boy who comes up and brings word of officer on watch says "In a few minutes expect to sight Hatteras light" which we do in an hour or so.

Now that we are fully on our journey and as yet unknown to us will give a general description of our little steamer, crew, etc. As I have stated the *Pocahontas* is a brig rigged screw steamer of 700 tons and rated at time of sailing 2nd class sloop of war. She is armed with six guns one one hundred rifled cannon one 32 rifle on fore castle and 4 32 broadsides guns. Her full complement of men should have been 150 but on account of the scarcity of seamen and the large number of boats in service she fell off largely from that number and at time of dont think we had much over 100 men. Such a variety of men could have hardly been scraped up for any other purpose. While there were a sprinkling of a few good sailors the many are a set of men who have followed boating on the canal. Some according to their own accounts have never been on a sail vessel and yet they have shipped as ordinary seamen.

The officers soon found out their short coming so frequent shifts take place both in gunnery and seamanship and in a few days there was an apparent change in the affairs on board. Our

19. Captain's clerk Perry Crombarger, Officers List.

officers cant say much for their ability as I am not competent to judge. Our Captain M. P. Jones is entirely a different man from what I should expect to find in an officer in such a charge. I don't think we have been favored with even one or two glimpses of him. He seems to be fond of his cabin; fat and gouty. The lieutenant of the ship seems to be quite a different man and you can see him busy at all times trying to make things more aright.

Our ship a few days before I joined her was to have a roving commission and was commanded by Davidson Phenix[20] who was quite a dark [two words erased by Dodson] this death placed M. P. Jones in command and from the way things looks the many departments seem to have changed their minds and the way we are steering seem to point to the monotony of an assistant in the blockade squadron Quite a change from what was expected as our thoughts were the "wide wide world."

Our knowing friend whose kind offer to plan things for our comfort and [———] we awaited ourselves of tells us to-day of the things he has bought all tinware mess pork beans etc and I tell you all are much out of humor. One barrel of pork we had to throw overboard. We were badly sold and he is disposed of his position. A masters mate tries his hand and we hope to fare a little better.

In our mess are the yeoman, capt clerk, paymaster clerk (the long Yankee), four masters mates and myself. Have quite a pleasant place to eat and rooms to occupy if we desire and everything goes in smoothly so far.

In the engineers department are one chief and 4 assistant engineers. Among the latter is Rodney Carter. Whenever we can get with one another we are sure to have a pleasant time. To

20. Dawson Phenix was a Naval Academy graduate and a lieutenant commander in 1862. He died February 20, 1864, shortly before the *Pocahontas* was to return to active duty. Callahan, *List of Officers*.

explain my own position on board is quite an undertaking. When I first joined the Navy thought from all the regiment of the surgeon who examined me certainly I am at least respectible connected in the service but when the first muster was called and I examined the grades I found out that there is a group of 1st class petty officers on board some being appointed as in my case head the list. My duties are put as a clerk in the drug store and when the sick call is over the balance of the time we do nothing. Our surgeon would write the prescription nurse wold bring it to the Dispensary to have me compound it. That was my duties and nothing more. Finding that there was a difference officially from my position and that occupied by the officers I made up my mind to keep my place and go through with a good grace and all of the wardroom officers who desired my company must come to me. I must say in justice to all that all barriors were thrown down and soon [————] I was made [to feel] if the government had failed to make any provisions all on board made me welcome and will add I never experienced the slightest slight or reference to position in any way but on the contrary was very often sent for and asked to spend my time with them. Even our captain would occasionally send that I should spend a few hours in his cabin.[21]

21. Dodson was obviously disappointed at his rating, which he explains at some length with emphasis on being treated as an equal by the ship's officers. His appointment was to the position of surgeon's steward, also called apothecary and referred to by the crew as "pills." What he actually did, especially when serving as Surgeon's Steward in charge of the Medical Department, was more like a present-day physician's assistant.

The status of the Civil War surgeon's steward is unclear. Rebecca Livingston, Naval Archivist at the National Archives, believes it was neither officer nor petty officer. On the *Pocahontas* muster rolls, Dodson is sometimes listed with the officers, sometimes with the crew. He probably wore the frock coat and visored cap worn by officers. His comment on December 8, 1864, concerning the buttons on his jacket tends to confirm this. See Hamersly, *A Naval Encyclopedia,* 38; Francis A. Lord, *Civil War Collector's Encyclopedia*

One of our principal amusements was for Dr, Pay Master, Carter and Mr Chandeler[22] to gather and reherse our pieces which we used on the Quarter Deck during Divine Service. Our Captain requests that we keep up our singing for the Sunday service. Our "Knowing Friend" Barnes as we call him was the jest of all and will give him credit for always preserving and even disposition. He is one of the poorest shaped men I have ever seen, very tall, stooping, firey red mustache which he would give an occasional twist when some dry joke was sure to follow. Think Barnes is on the make at all times and generally had an eye to business. He was in just such a position where he could turn all things to account. Being with the Pay Master Department he had all the accounts to keep & stores to [——————] which gave him a grand field for speculation if it ever presented the opportunity.

While the constant daily exercises of guns at quarters was going on there was a lack of a commander of one division. Barnes, being awkward himself, here made a strive for glory. It seems he got command of the awkward squad For such a farce officered by such a figure as Barnes made with a sort of sack coat flapping in the wind could only been called by such a name. His figure and tones of voice as he repeated the orders from the Quarter Deck made such mirth.

"Run in: run out Toney Tucker[23] what are you about" which was the only thing that ever seemed to raise any of his ire (Toney was an odd genius, black as ink, a perfect baboon and it had

(New York: Castle Books, by arrangement with Stackpole Books, 1965), 325. Dodson's uniform probably closely resembled that of the carpenter's mate shown in the photograph on page 319, except for the insignia.

22. Mr. Chandeler was Joseph W. Chandler, Acting Ensign (Officers List).

23. Toney Tucker was Anthony Tucker, Landsman, "Muster Roll of Crew of USS *Pocahontas,* April 1, 1864," manuscript, Record Group 24, National Archives. Hereafter cited as Crew's List.

fallen to Barnes' lot to have him as powder boy). Barnes for some time could be seen with his book "Ward on Broadside Guns" trying to pick up but soon he had such fun poked at him as to give up his Division. I suppose had his gun been close to the captain's quarters and he would have observed the fun the idlers were engaged in at times of quarters certainly he never would have permitted such a farce.

Our Pay Master[24] is a good sort of fellow rather effeminate looking though he seemed to be a regular . . . man. He was exceedingly kind to me. Dr Mann appears already as a friend. Every day finds us together after sick call. He is a fine looking man. Unfortunately he has a failing. Will use too much stimulation. Have had a long conversation with him. I had since joining the Navy upon special occasions met his wife who had told me her great trouble. She is from Troy New York. She asked me "when I get him by himself to speak to him about his failing." Dr and I have just come from the fore top and have had a long chat. He has promised to send every drop of his private stock of wines and liquors and give them to my care to be locked in the Dispensary. Says "Don't you remember the day you first called to see me. I offered you wine and insisted. My wife was in the adjoining room and observed saw and heard us. As soon as I was through asking you questions and went out she says "Doctor you take that young man." So the advise from his wife was the cause of his change of mind.

One quite agreeable fellow is Barney Duvell[25] quite a songster he used to get up some fun by his spirited songs and we often gave him credit for getting up the song that insulted Barnes the Yankee who attempted to manage a gun division astern.

24. The Paymaster was Acting Paymaster A. J. Wright Jr. (Officer's List).
25. I was unable to identify Barney Duvell.

April 19

On the ocean pleasantly steaming til 4 PM. The wind is blowing quite hard and we are so close to Hatteras and things look too much like a storm that all things are "made snug." Storm sails are set and everything ready for the blow which came at six. The Pocahontas seems to be a good sea boat for though we are jumping around lively she is quite dry. They say this is a storm but I have seen it equally rough on the Chesapeake Bay.

April 20

To-day storm abated. Heavy roll for part of the morning. Later in the day made an offing. Made signal for a pilot. Received one and sailed into Port Royal.

April 21

Lying in harbor of Port Royal. There is a large fleet of vessels at this place. Took in a supply of coal. Sent home letters. Only stayed til night when we sailed out of the harbor.

22 & 23

Spent these days on the ocean sailing by the coast of Georgia and Florida. The ocean is quite smooth. We are not subjected to the rolling of the ship as several days ago. We are steaming along quietly.

24 25 26 April

A Sunday. Heavy head winds. Above days almost a stand still butting the waves. One large billow came dashing its spray on our bows & gave us our first sprinkling added to our slow progress. Was raining most of the time and quite uncomfortable on deck.

April 27

On the ocean. A clear day. All the sailors are drying cloths and it looks like a wash day on shore. First time I ever saw flying fish. Seemed quite curious to us all. Also saw Nautalus. They would spread out their web sails and really look like a miniature craft under way.

April 28

Passing the island of Abaco. Saw the noted "Hole in the Wall." What a beautiful appearance the small island of Eluthera presented as it seemed to rise up from the water later in the evening. So green looked like a perfect gem. Some of the inhabitants came off to sell fruit but our steamer did not stop and we soon left them all behind. Their little boats seemed to be frail structures a sort of dug out canoes.[26]

29th of April

Going over the Bahama Banks. Some of the sailors told us if we would go aloft and look we should have a much grander sight. We did so and 'tis surprising as [————] of the fore top what a clear view one has. The water was very clear and we could see the smallest objects on the bottom. Such a variety of marine plants of bright colors star fish sea grass etc make quite a variety.

30th

This was a fine day and as there was no one sick the Dr and I were soon up the fore top where we spent most of the day

26. Little and Great Abaco are the northernmost of the islands in the Bahamas and would have been the first seen by Dodson. Eleuthera, also mentioned by him, is directly south of the Abacos.

The Hole in the Wall is a lighthouse complex on the extreme southern tip of the Abacos. The lighthouse, now automated and unmanned, is currently the home of the Bahamas Marine Mammal Survey, which records sightings of whales and dolphins in Bahamian waters.

reading with an occasional look at some interesting thing strange fish and birds that came close to the steamer. To-day could not eat any dinner. We had beans soup and I dont like it though for supper our cook tells me he has saved me my share and will bake them. They are good.

May 1, 1864

We arrived at Key West Sunday. Had service with singing. At noon in company with several friends went on shore. We took a long walk into interior. How hot the sun seems at this place. Suppose the sandy soil has very little to cool off the rays. In the town we find quite an amount of business[,] quite a station of vessels, supplys, coal, etc. During our walk through the island we came to really a friendly home. Twas cozy and offered to us quite a retreat from the heat that beams on us so fiercely. The owner was a colored man who made us welcome and gave us limes juice as a drink a sort of lemonade. Found it quite refreshing. All seemed highly delighted with our trip which occupied our time until quite late in the afternoon. Returning to the ship found her at the wharf getting ready to "coal up" on the morrow.

May 2nd Key West

Coaling ship quite a dirty job to get clear of the dust etc. Went up town a little while. Sat in front of one of the hotels and did not make much of an effort to fancy one in a tropical town. Saw plenty of banana fruit, limes, pineapples, etc. Then the little donkeys. 'Twas amazing to see some of the sailors try to ride them. Go for a few rods & then of a sudden stop and with a bow he let his rider over his head. Turns around with [———] and returns to his stable. Went around the wharf later in the day. A large number of steamers are in port. The noted Slaver *Wanderer* [27]

27. Originally a rich man's yacht, the *Wanderer* changed ownership, was refitted as a slaver, and delivered a human cargo of Congolese to Jekyl Island,

lay close to us. She is a queer looking craft and I am told queer looking scences have been enacted on her decks. Several steamers come in bringing prizes.

May 3rd

After coaling ship we started. Could not go over the bar. Came back and waited for flood tide which occured at 8 PM. We soon started afresh and such good speed many sails and steam. Late at night saw a steamer which from signal made out to be the *"Massachusetts"* the one Charles Blades is on. I learn subsequently that Charlie fell down the hol[d] of this vessel in a storm and disabled him so as to cause his return home.

May 4th

It has been stated by some of the officers that our destination is New Orleans and from the way we are sailing think they are right. Blowing hard, a sail reported we bear down upon her. Soon bring her to by a shot across her bow. Checked papers and allowed her to sail on.

Georgia, in November 1858. Later she was stolen from her owners by the ship's captain, who embarked on a voyage of slaving and piracy. The crew mutinied, left him at sea in a small boat, and delivered up the vessel to the authorities in Boston on Christmas Eve 1859.

Complex criminal and civil proceedings brought no convictions and, under southern registry, *Wanderer* was confiscated at Key West, Florida, when Federal forces occupied that place. In May 1863 she was formally incorporated into the U.S. Navy, served as a water carrier and supply ship, and captured several Confederate merchantmen. Refitted as a hospital ship, *Wanderer* was at Key West in May 1864, where Dodson saw her. Two months later her entire crew came down with yellow fever. After the war she served as a merchantman and sank off Cuba in 1871. *Dictionary of American Naval Fighting Ships,* 8:90–91. Tom Henderson Wells, *The Slave Ship Wanderer* (Athens: University of Georgia Press, 1967), makes fascinating reading.

5th On the Gulf of Mexico

Strong wind and we are sailing very fast. Sea running very high. Cant walk on deck without an occasional slip. Dr says can we stand the roll up the cross ties. We are here and dont find it so very difficult after we are once snugly fixed there.

6 On the Gulf of Mexico

Late in the evening we come to muddy water and in a short time make the passes of the Mississippi River. Though the sea is so rough 'tis astonishing how easily we took on a pilot and with what speed he came on board is surprising. The water here is very muddy like a mountain stream when a freshlet occurs.

May 7

After having been tossed upon the Gulf so violently during our trip from Key West the change is quite comfortable. Seems so quiet moving along the narrow stream and this muddy flow of water is the famous Mississippi that we have heard so much about.

May 8

Coming on deck find the ship anchored off quarintine. There are several vessels flying the "Yellow Flag." We have several cases of fever on board. There is grave fears we are about to be detained. The sick man was a master's mate Mr. Duncan. He was one of our party that took the stroll through Key West and ever since he has been confined to his bed. He is particularly cross and particularly so to nurse Randall[28] who reports him not satisfied with anything he does for him.

28. Randall was Abraham Randall, landsman and nurse on *Pocahontas* crew lists of April 1 and July 1, 1864. Crew's List. Mr. Duncan was Acting Masters Mate John W. Duncan. Callahan, *List of Officers*.

May 9

In quarintine some miles below New Orleans. While here we have good chance to see the result of a portion of the fight Farragut had upon his approach to New Orleans. Find several old wrecks, rams, etc. Also see the damage to the trees. 'Tis quite plain the mark where broadsides plowed through the woods and left wide gaps.[29] The steamer winds up anchor and we are en route for the city.

May 10th

Steaming up the Mississippi. One moment we run close enough to jump out on the bank, occasionally passing a little hamlet, a plantation. Alligators are quite abundant. One old fellow did not seem ill at ease when, fastened on an old log, we ran quite close to him. At 2 PM we came to the city. Suppose we will spend some time here as they say the boilers are to be overhauled.

May 11th

Coaled the ship. Suddenly no one among our mess can tell while at breakfast why this early move and unusual stir overhead. A rumor we are to go down the coast and engage in some kind of expedition. Of course we do not hear or know anything. So far

29. Realizing the strategic and commercial importance of New Orleans, a joint army-navy expedition was organized in late 1861 to take the city. General Benjamin F. Butler led the army contingent, Admiral David G. Farragut the navy. Farragut successfully ran past Forts Jackson and Saint Philip south of New Orleans without loss and destroyed the small Confederate fleet defending it as Butler approached from the east. Farragut captured the city April 25, 1862. The forts surrendered four days later. Butler's troops then occupied the city, and he applied a harsh but efficient rule over it. New Orleans remained in Federal hands for the rest of the war and became the base for the West Gulf Blockading Squadron to which Dodson's ship belonged. He will write of it often. Mark M. Boatner III, *The Civil War Dictionary* (1959; New York: Vintage Civil War Library, 1991), 591–92.

one thing: vessels just coming into port dont have such stir and bustle as is here today. So something is up sure.

May 12

In the company of two other steamers we are steaming down the river. It seems at some place on the coast the Confederates had captured two of our steamers and have grown a little encouraged and [it is] supposed at any time will make some sort of attack on the Gulf. We spoke several vessels who gave us a rather gloomy acct of things. Says "There was quite a fleet and large force of Confederates at the place" but we are heading for the place and everthing wears a war like appearance. Guns are loaded with shell.

May 13

Came to Pass Calcasu Eastling.[30] We saw the Confederate steamers inside the bay behind a neck of land. Our captain being senior we became the flag ship. At 10 AM the *Pocahontas* led the way, the other steamers supporting us. Soon as we got into position we opened fire from our hundred pounder and it soon was apparent the range was good for the steamers did not long expose themselves but moved further up the bay. On account of the shallow water on the bar there was no pursuit and all hovered off for consultation. Our consorts in this was the *New London* and another steamer *Aroostic*.[31] A boat from *New London* went on shore to look at things during the night and were captured.

---

30. Pass Calcasieu, Louisiana, is on the Gulf of Mexico about fifty miles west of the Louisiana-Texas border. Dodson referred to it frequently with various spellings.

31. USS *New London* was a small (221-ton), wooden, screw steamer, number of guns varies. OR:II:1:159.

USS *Aroostock*, 597 tons, was a wood screw steamer, number of guns varies. She was sold by the government in Hong Kong in 1869. OR:II:1:39.

May 14

Laying off the Pass. Plain view of works and vessels of the Confederates. During yesterday's firing I asked doctor's permission to leave my quarters which in time of action is below decks. He gave it to me I went up to the fore top only keeping as much out of sight of officers on deck as possible. There I had a good chance to see where the heavy shots would strike around. The steamers took a splash. Sometimes a shell would be given them and its explosion would make quite a stir among the boats. Seems we had come to a stand still and quit firing. The captain sent for me and asked if I knew what danger I had exposed myself [to]. While we were steaming over the bar had we struck bottom the speed we had up would have broken our mast.

May 15

We received orders to sail for New Orleans. Left several vessels to blockade the Pass. Started at night.

May 16

Spoke the *Agusta Dinsmore* quite early in the morning. She came near running into us. Sailed in the Mississippi River. Our expedition had been a little change though cant see how anyway how good was done as it seems we had left the place without the slightest resistence on part of the Confederates. I suppose the Department thought the place not of sufficient importance to take and hold. Prepared to have a good blockade.

May 17

Arrived at New Orleans. Spent portion of the day writing letters. At night troubled with the various kinds of insects mosquitos etc.

May 18

Off New Orleans. Mr Duncan is quite sick. In fact we have kept him on board only because of our sudden departure from this place last week. One of our men deserted while our cutter was ashore. They captured him the following day and at time of writing he is in irons.

May 19

Mr Cromburger and I have enjoyed a trip through the city. Am much amused at the cars and horses they use in this Section. A mule seems to be the motive power. Have no conductors. You deposit your fare in box which could be a piece of cardboard or any other little thing you happen to have in your pocket. The city has beautiful streets [with] double row of trees and to us who have such narrow streets the change is very much admired. Certainly this city with its abundent room should be a healthy one and could hardly conceive how such dreadful diseases should ever have been known here.

May 20 & 21

Off New Orleans. Remained most of the time down on the berth deck. Received a letter from Clay dated the day I started from Phila containing news of C A F conduct. One case of high fever on board. Dr Mann quite ill today (21st). One case had to use the lancet on his thumb which gave him much relief. He had been suffering so long from a gathering which could not be drawn by any kind of poulice so sought but to relieve him.

22 May

Went on shore for a short time. Close to shore lay a big Mississippi steamer converted into a floating hospital. Was full of wounded at this time as Banks had just met disaster on the Red

River[32] and many of the wounded were on this steamer. She had excellent quarters and fitted up in the most elaborate manner. I found in her a beautiful little drug store or dispensary and three druggists were assigned to her.

I had quite an agreeable surprise while on board. She was the fleet surgeon's of the Upper Mississippi floating hospital Dr Niman Pinckeny from my own county. I sent him my card and he gave me quite a welcome. He thought I had come to join him as he had written to Purser Hambleton to have me come out. He was quite surprised when I pointed to the *Pochontas* and told him I belonged to her (I had sailed before his letter had reached St. Michaels). The Dr, after showing me the fine sanitary points this steamer presented, showed me quite a number of the wounded of which there were all sorts. Getting late said good bye. Just as I was coming off the large gang board of the steamer fell. Killed a young man who was under it.

From the 23rd to the 28th of May

Off New Orleans. They are giving the machines an overhauling and on deck there is no comfort so much of the time spent on the berth deck. Not much pleasure going on shore as we dont know anyone. On the night of the 27th we had a large fire commenced on the levee. Before it was over eight steamers were consumed. During the fire awful explosions took place. T'was a fearfully grand sight.

32. Because of the French threat in Mexico the Lincoln administration desired a presence in Texas. To achieve this a joint army-navy expedition under General Nathaniel P. Banks and Admiral David D. Porter was planned to penetrate up the Red River into Texas. The campaign was a failure, and it was only with heavy fighting and skilled engineering to overcome river obstacles that the Federal forces made their withdrawal with considerable loss in men and ships. Boatner, *Civil War Dictionary*, 635–39.

The physician from Talbot County, Maryland, was Dr. Ninian Pinkney, a career naval officer who rose from assistant surgeon in 1841 to medical director in 1871. He died six years later. Callahan, *List of Officers*.

May 28th

On board *Pocahontas*. Mr McLeery[33] "Acting Ensign" was ordered to gunboat No 48 as executive officer. He did not seem at all disturbed when he found he was to leave our ship.

May 29–30–31

Off New Orleans. Several men got into a fight and several are now in irons. On the 31st took Nurse Randall went to Erata Street Hospital and got full supply of medicine. Later in the day took a trip to Lake Ponchutrain.[34]

June 1st

There is a large number of vessels in port also a French Man of War. One of the larger Mississippi River steamers just past. They are curious. So much upper works and such front hulls.

June 2nd

Hauled into the levee. Took a supply of coal. The anchor could not be taken in so we had to cut the chain so lost it. Mr Duncan has not been himself since we took the stroll through Key West so Dr concludes to have him sent so he is carried to the steamer "Admiral" and sails for his home. Nurse Randall gives a sigh of relief when he went for using his own words "he was the most *troublement* man he ever saw."

June 3rd

Sailing upon the Mississippi. Soon upon the Gulf of Mexico. On the 4th arrived at Pass Calachu the scene of our last exploits.

---

33. Acting Ensign Thomas McLeary. Callahan, *List of Officers*.
34. Pontchartrain is a large lake with a narrow outlet to the Gulf of Mexico near the Louisiana-Mississippi border. New Orleans lies along its southeast shoreline.

Found the gunboat *New London* still there. During the day a very large number of fish around the ship.

On the 5th arrived off Galveston.[35] Found quite a large fleet there doing blockade. Several sailors went fishing from our steamer. Caught several young sharks.

35. Galveston, Texas had been taken by Federal forces in 1862, recaptured by the Confederates in 1863, and held until the end of the war.

West Gulf Blockading Squadron
JUNE 4, 1864 – OCTOBER 7, 1864

June 6

Off Galveston. At night ran close to the shore. Took our station in the blockading squadron. Fired upon by the forts. At an early hour weighed anchor and started for Brazos River.[36] Made the pass late at night.

June 8th

On the alert off Brazos Expecting the *Harriet Lane*[37] which they say was seen "hovering around." News came that since we left Galveston two blockade runners had succeeded in running into that port.

June 9, 10, 11

Off Brazos. Had rather a pleasant surprise on the 10th. Supply steamer came down. We had fresh provisions and ice for two or three days. On the 11th we sailed close to rebel's works. Their cavalry are scouting around the coast.

June 12 1864

Left Brazos. Came to Galveston. Ran close to the forts. Received few shots from one of them. Hauled off as storm was threatening and came to anchor.

June 13th

Strong gale blowing. One of the fleet lost her masts close to us.

36. The Brazos River is about fifty miles south of Galveston, Texas.

37. The *Harriet Lane* was a former Union ship captured by the Confederates at Galveston in January 1863, when they retook the city. She was a 619-ton wood, side wheel steamer, armed with six guns, that was converted into a blockade runner at Havana, Cuba, at the war's end. *OR*:II:1:256. Dodson also mentions her on August 26, 1864.

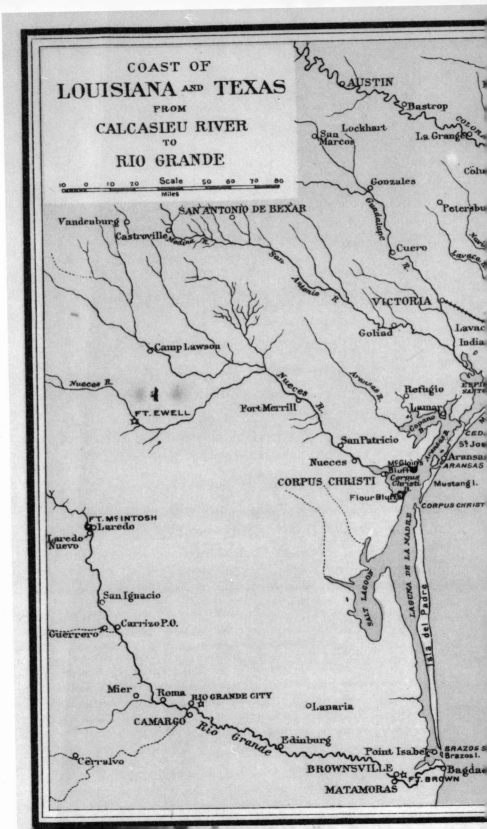

COAST OF
LOUISIANA AND TEXAS
FROM
CALCASIEU RIVER
TO
RIO GRANDE

Scale
10   0   10   20   50   60   70   80
Miles

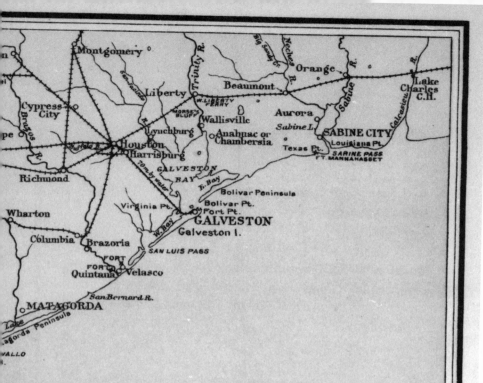

GULF OF MEXICO

(*From* Official Records of the Union and Confederate
Navies in the War of the Rebellion *(Washington,
D.C.: Government Printing Office, 1894).*)

We keep a vigilant watch for upon such evenings as this the blockade runners try to run past and Galveston is quite a desirable port for them to reach.

June 14

In the middle of the day calmed down. We went alongside of a brig and took on coal.

June 15th

Sailed from off Galveston and came to Sabine Pass.[38] One of the steamers doing blockade at this place had on board Dr Mann's brother[39] as "Paymaster." He called to see the Dr at night. Had a rehearsal of choir.

16th

Off Pass Sabine. Pleasant weather. The watch off are amusing themselves fishing. Dr and I have tried our hands. One of the men caught a young shark. Twas a good flavor as we all enjoyed a piece of him.

17th to 24th

Off Pass Sabine. Some days very rainy during which time I spent it under decks. We had frequent rehearsals of choir and managed to pass the time as pleasantly as possible. Randall our nurse is a quiet colored man and has to meet the jeers of the men because

38. Pass Sabine is on the Texas-Louisiana border where the Sabine River flows into the Gulf of Mexico. The river divides the two states. The *Pocahontas* often did blockade duty there.

39. Dr. Mann's brother, Acting Assistant Paymaster William A. Mann, entered the service August 20, 1862, and was mustered out January 1, 1866. Callahan, *List of Officers*. He served on the USS *Cayuga* at this time. Department of the Navy, "Navy Historical Center" web site, June 12, 1998, Officers of Navy Yards, Shore Stations and Vessels, January 1, 1865, West Gulf Blockading Squadron. Other citations from this source are as above and will be referred to hereafter as NHC.

he does nothing. Of course when there is no sickness He had an easy time. He is a tailor by trade. This week he made me a pair of flannel pants — unsatisfactory.

On the 24th it seemed Randall would have something to do for there was an unusually long sick list but perhaps some of them were sham[m]ing for the next day was one of such activity on board and perhaps they got wind of it. A general wholesale cleaning day on ship.

June 25 & 26

Pass Sabine. What a time on the 25th. So much scrubbing and washing one cant find a place to rest unless the throwing of water and the grinding sound of "holey stones" are heard.[40] So I keep to the main top and certainly they will not require this place to be disturbed but soon several lads came up and had to open an old box to examine it. Found the captain had ordered to be kept there and we soon left this place. On the 26th Sunday rest divine service performed by captain. Choir sang.

June 27

Off Sabine. At 4 PM steamer reported. Proved to be the mail boat. Received letters from father and mother and I tell you they were welcome. Having chance sent letter north.

Called up early on the 28th. Found we had a sick officer. Also found we were steaming quite fast to some point. Soon made Pass Calcasiau running in as far as the draught of the vessel would permit. Commenced throwing shell at the Confederate steamers. Soon as we got in range and position the *USS Cayuga*[41]

40. The holy stone was a sandstone used to scrub decks. There are various explanations of how it got its name, two of which are that it was used most often on Sundays and that the men knelt while using it. Hamersly, *A Naval Encyclopedia,* 346.

41. USS *Cayuga* was a 507-ton wood, screw steamer, number of guns varied. *OR*:II:1:53–54. When he again mentions her, Dodson calls her the *Cunoga.*

took a position on our right. We commenced firing. Kept it up a little while then broke off. Consultation followed and we did not return to the work anymore. At night we sailed for Pass Sabine.

June 29th

Came to Pass Sabine anchored. We can slip our cables in a minute with a device to buoy them up. Early that morning a small object was seen at starboard. A cutter was lowered and sent. Proved to be a Texas reffugee. He had rowed out too far during the night and when came on board was much grateful and desired to remain on board. Today we treated under flag of truce with the Confederates.

30th June

Tonight a boat is manned by 10 men under charge of master's mate Gould[42] and sent in close to shore as picket duty with such instructions as giving signals, etc. She puts off and is soon lost in the darkness. Looks as a lonely trip taken in such a small craft.

June 31

Off Pass Sabine. Picket boat returned. For neglecting some duty the officer in charge was placed under arrest. Seemed to have taken the young man down very much. In his desire to do much he had failed to obey his orders.

July 1, 1864

This month came upon [us] and finds good weather. Sea smooth and everything going on pleasantly. In the afternoon tried to get the choir to sing old Antioch. Dr and Paymaster our heavy bass

42. Mr. Gould was Masters Mate James L. Gould. The transgression for which he was arrested must not have been too serious because he was promoted to acting ensign on May 3, 1865, and mustered out March 19, 1866. Callahan, *List of Officers;* NHC.

46

will insist that either one or the other comes in too soon and tis amusing to hear their retorts. At night the steamer *Cynoga* came and took her position close to us.

July 2

Day past as usual. At 8 PM a picket boat was sent close to shore. At 11 PM a light reported on port bow. Supposing it to be a blockade runner a hasty order to up anchor. Captain's clerk and [I] were sitting on the gun carriage. He says "lets help." We flew to the capstan soon found we were no good as the sailors had the best of us having practice. We were glad to get away and then w[e] received a few blows. I had on slippers and they never accounted any good afterwards. After we had steamed out a considerable distance lost the sight of light. We returned to our station at 2 AM. We had a little change at any rate and a little sea breeze.

July 3rd

Sabbath all hands to muster divine service. Choir sang some old pieces on the Quarter deck. Today we have a beautiful scene bef[ore] and around us the sun for a few minutes gets to shine and the glow is beautiful. On one side as far as the eye can see is the Gulf of Mexico looking like a mirror, so smooth at this time. I[n] front of us is the steamer "*Estrella*,"[43] a side wheel boat was captured and converted into a gunboat. Even the low lands of Texas and La seem to show off to an advantage this evening. Everyone who understands how softening is the effect of such a sunset as we have would surely understand why everything seem so unusually beautiful and so much appreciated. I shall always remember this one sunset off Texas.

43. USS *Estrella,* an armed 435-ton side wheel steamer, was transferred in 1862 from the army. *OR*:II:1:80

July 4th

Observed as much of a holiday as possible. Work suspended Flag and streamers flying.

July 5th & 6th

Off Sabine Pass. Spent these days variously engaged. We would go aloft and while there a game of checkers, a nap, and talk of w[hen] we all get home again. Dr Mann used to come up with us and give quite an account of his being in one of the assaults upon Fort Sumpter.

July 7th

The steamer *Bermuda* came direct from Philadelphia with supplies of fresh provisions so for a day or so we would far much better. A few of us came out of the mess and concluded to live on ships provisions. Cadmus, Dozell and myself.[44] We have a cook for our mess. Small as it is we are more comfortable fixed than [when] we messed with so many as there always seemed to be some disagreement.

July 8 1864

Off Pass Sabine. Steamer *Estrella* left us for Pensacola. The USS *Arizona* came up to fill her place. Tonight went in close to shore to act as picket boat.

July 9th 1864

Mr Cromberger tells me he is to be sent home in the *Bermuda* upon her return North. He was Captain's clerk but soon as our ship did not rate high enough to give Barnes his position I think

44. Cadmus was Yeoman James C. Cadmus, crew's list, July 1, 1864. Dodson later identifies Cadmus as the ship's yeoman in his entry for July 22, 1864. I was unable to identify Dozell.

it was determined for Barnes to act for the Paymaster though he would receive appointment as Captain's clerk hence the change.

July 10th

Sunday morning service on deck. *Bermuda* arrived. Mr Cromberger left on her. He was much pleased to go as he was quite tired of the blockade.

From the 11th to the 20th

Off Sabine Pass. We were favored with a mail boat one day and soon afterward a supply steamer came around. Received five letters from home folks. Also a good supply of fresh beef. I missed Mr Cromberger very much. However Dr used to come up and spend much time with me. During one visit we went up the fore top and while there Dr commenced conversation. Wanted to quit the life he was leading change and become a better man as he expressed it. Wanted to know if I would go to "Troy"[45] and engage in drug business with him. Also stated that he would revoke my appointment if I decided and resign himself.

Poor Dr he has had a strain on him and from his actions I find he must be much alarmed at his symptoms. Says to me one day if anything happens to me cut me up and place me in a barrel of tar as I have a dread of being cast in the sea. Poor Dr how much confidence you seem to place in me. I do hope no such thing will be.

He would grow quite melancholy some days and at such times seemed to desire to be in the Dispensary with me or at the fore top. He was exceedingly kind to me and always treated me with much respect.

One day he seemed quite cheerful. We spent a long time

45. Dodson earlier referred to Troy, New York, as Mrs. Mann's home. Dr. Mann's comment "if anything happens to me" was prescient as Dodson's entries on subsequent days will reveal.

tracking down the water we used on board. Suspected something not right as many of the men were troubled after drinking. Found trace of copper which led to examination of retort and found the cure. (We all at sea use the ocean water condensed.)

20 July

Fresh breezes. Dr Mann taken sick turns over the medical department to me. Two cases of Ferenailes. Applied lancet.[46]

July 21

Sail reported. Soon all is astir on board as she bears on so boldly are ready to receive her friend or foe. Proves to be the USS *Agusta Dinsmore*. I went on board. Delivered a sick man to be sent to New Orleans hospital. The Texan refugee went on board soon after.

22 & 23

Dr Mann remains on sick list. Cadmus our yeoman went home on the *Admiral* for Philadelphia. Our captain sends word for me to come see him. Found him with his large limbs placed on a chair. He was full of boils[47] and ready to boil over as his cabin boy had just hurt him by letting a [————] fall upon his foot. Fixed him up with flaxseed poulices etc.

July 24

Off Sabine Pass. A flag of truce received on board. Captain of the

---

46. Ferenailes may refer to Fereol's nodes, subcutaneous nodes or swellings that sometimes occur in acute rheumatism. A lancet is a small surgical knife.

47. Boils are painful nodules of circumscribed inflammation caused by *staphylococci*. Flaxseed is linseed, a dried seed of *Linum usitatissimum* used to soothe irritation and soften skin. Poultices are cloth and a moist mass applied to a given area.

Morning Light[48] captured a year ago, captured on the coast. He had been a pirate.

25

Rehearsed choir in the evening. Capt seemed to enjoy the singing and requested his rooms to be kept open

26 July

Captain M P Jones our commander sends for me. Says he is affected very much and did one see him they would think him a sort of Job so many boils on him. Well we talked and during the conversation asked what I thought of Dr Mann as he had noticed his actions and had thought them strange. While I was fully impressed with the fact that Dr was entirely unfit for duty I did not think proper to give my full opinion as it would come to his ear and perhaps make a coolness between us.

July 27

Off Sabine Pass. Gulf rough. We are much closer to shore than is comfortable as far as sea room is concerned but close to the mouth of the pass lay a large rebel steamer. She is what is called cotton clad. Bales of it are placed around her sides and from her formible look we may expect some exciting sport if she attempts to come out.

28

Still on alert for the steamer. Our fires are up and everything ready.

29

Wind blowing. Alarm bell rings out. Soon cry of fire and in a

48. USS *Morning Light,* a 938-ton sailing ship of eight guns, was captured off Sabine Pass on January 31, 1863. *OR*:II:1:51.

short time the fore part of our ship was in a dense smoke. After much exertion and stir fire was extinguished. Came near choking us so dense was the smoke in the berth deck.

30 & 31

Still off the Pass. Dr very sick fortunately not many of the crew. Steamer *Arizona* sailed from here to Calcasieu Pass.

August 1st to 5th

Hot times not much air stiring. We had the deck washed down frequently which went far towards making things more comfortable.

Aug 5

A small cutter left our ship and rowed toward the shore. Went as far as the wreck of the *Clifton*.[49] Under flag to truce received some women who had permission to return to New Orleans. At 3 PM the *Arkansas* came up brought a mail for us.

6, 7 & 8 August

Very little of note occured the above days. Our lives presented the same routine as the previous days. On the 8th Dr Mann was taken quite ill. Found him suffering much. Seems to be a difficulty in his circulation. Paymaster and I takes our first watch beside his cot. Have the Dr rubbed well with a little distilled spirits. Seems to give him a little relief for he slept the last portion of the night.

Aug 9th

Our captain signals for the surgeons of the fleet to come on

49. This *Clifton* was an 892-ton side wheel steamer with a varying number of guns. She surrendered to the Confederates at Sabine Pass on September 8, 1863. Another *Clifton* was later named USS *Shokoken*. OR:I:2:59, 208.

board. They consulted and concluded Dr Mann should be sent home first chance. We had the Dr placed in cot which is hung under the poop deck. Randall nurse will now have the care of constant attention to him. Medical Department turned over to me. Fortunately there are very little ailments among the men.

10

Three cutters go into the pass. Received several ladies and had them placed on board the *Arkansas*. Sent to New Orleans. All done under flag of truce.

11

Gulf rough. Dr from the US Steamer *Gertrude*[50] came today. Dr Mann requested that I tend to our few sick.

12

Very heavy wind. A boat from the shore with flag of truce sighted. She could not come out on account of the waves. Crew drilled at the broad side guns.

Aug 13

Dr Mann today is worse. He at times is quite unmanagable. He raves very much. Today wanted this morning to open an artery and would have perhaps inflicted some harm upon himself if I had not made Randall take knife away. Paymaster Mann, Dr Mann's brother, came up to see him today from his ship which lay at Calcasieu. Now it is necessary for one of the surgeons to come and see Dr Mann every day. They do all in their power but between them I am afraid they allow Dr too much opiates.

---

50. USS *Gertrude* was a 350-ton iron screw steamer, eight guns. She was captured November 16, 1863, by the USS *Vanderbilt* off Eleuthera in the Bahamas and was purchased by the government from the New York Prize Court. *OR*:II:1:95.

14

Off Sabine. We had a little scare. Saw several small objects floating. Thought some infernal machines been sent out to us. Found to be a keg and a jug Thinking even these things meant mischief we had them shoved quietly by our steamer when they drifted to sea.

Aug 15th to 19th

Of course when one aboard is so ill there is much care and consideration to be exercised. During the first part of Dr troubles he thought it necessary to use liquors and up to the time of the other Dr calling to see him used it and morphine rather freely. When they came they found it necessary to restrict yet always allowed him enough and between them I am sure too much.

Poor Dr did not like my firm stand. After talking with our captain I had upon several occasions refused him his full demands for the liquor. I could not help but notice he was much taken up with Randall, or as he would call him "my good man Randall." Suspecting all not right I watched and found Randall was supplying him with whiskey from a bottle under the pillow. Randall was much alarmed. I can see that Dr is growing worse that only a matter of time before the end comes.

Aug 19th

Dr much prostrated though he seems a little rational today. Sent for me and would have me introduced afresh to all who stood around. Poor Dr his aim was no doubt well for under impulses he seemed he wanted to do something to attone for the ravings of the past week. We are now seated under the poop deck alongside the cot. He requested Randall to read a chapter in the Bible. Dr has conversation with his brother who continues on board. He spoke of his wife and child. 'Tis a very sad picture presented here this afternoon.

Silence is observed as far as possible and none of the heavy work if excess [————] is or has been [done] for several days. All have made up mind that Dr will not last much longer. We are all quite tired out watching and caring for him. This evening his random speech seems to point that he is not himself as he does not know us and is often engaged conversing with imaginary persons.

August 20, 1864

Dr Mann died at 2 AM. Short time before his death he was very quiet and collected. Seemed to have grown quite rational in conversing with his brother. Wanted us all to remain told him messages to take to his wife, child and parents just as composed as if he was doing an ordinary office of everyday life. Mr Mann bears up like a brave man but anyone can see in him grief of the deepest type.

Conversing with him found a hard thing to agree to have him thrown overboard. Of course my voice could not afford a protection to such stern measures but I should have supposed that had our commander used the slightest effort we certainly could have under flag of truce given him a place on land. I dont know much about the objections on either side but I think humanity would have overbalanced all objection.

Finding that the burial would be at sea 'twas appointed the Paymaster and myself should get things ready. We had Dr draped in full uniform sewed up in canvas and then the carpenter made a coffin and by 10 in the morning (6 hours after his death) he was in it. We then steamed out into the Gulf. We had holes bored into the coffin and when we had the Dr sewed up in canvas 4-32 pound shot were placed in with him two at the head and two at his feet.

Above and right: pages from Dodson's hymnal. (Maryland Historical Society.)

Our thoughts are quite sad as we contemplate [the] scene before us. Here we are steaming out to sea to find in its broad bosom a grave for our late surgeon and friend. All is still on board ship. Gulf, elements are all in full accord with our feelings and massive quiet seems to be around. The evening glow of the fast setting sun makes a solemn picture.

Suddenly the silence is broken when the Boatswain's call rings out "All hands bury dead." To a landsman this is fearful. I remember my feelings that evening. Have heard the same cry many times but not with such force did it come as upon this occasion.

When we had steamed out of sight of land and well out to sea the body was brought and placed on an incline plane. Captain Jones read the burial service and the body in coffin is raised then is slipped into the water. We thought there would be no difficulty in its sinking but when it struck the waves it seemed to almost leap back on the vessel on account of the coffin being so buoyant. The cutter was lowered, additional weights placed upon it then a few gurgling sounds and it sunk into the deep. Immediately after this sad performance we started for Calcasieu

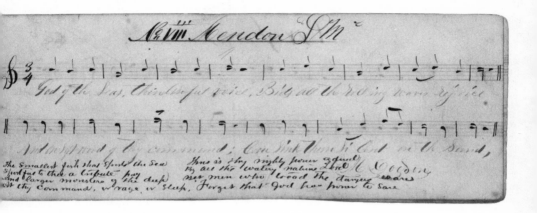

Pass to carry Drs brother to his ship stationed there. At midnight we came to the pass. The Paymaster bid us good bye and left us.

Aug 21st

Around Sabine Pass. This morning at sick call we can hardly express feelings. A ship's company liable a portion to be taken ill at any minute. Certainly here is a responsibility which I hope will soon be removed. During Dr's illness our quarterly report and papers had been neglected so had to get them up which is a new duty as he used to do this himself. Supply steamer arrived today bringing us a lot of medical stores I had ordered last quarter.

Sabbath duties observed at divine services on the quarter deck in the evening our choir took part last hymn words "Softly now the light of day fades upon my sight away" to the tune of *Hendon*.[51] Later in the evening called to ask captain (as I thought

51. "Hendon" was a tune written in the early part of the nineteenth century by Henri Abraham Cesar Malan, a Swiss preacher and hymn writer who also composed the melodies for most of his hymns. It is believed he named it after a village in England where he once lived. It was quite popular in evangelical circles in the United States. Dodson used it with two

best) to have one of the surgeons from our fleet to come on board occasionally and he had agreed to do so. Fortunately I am well acquainted with Dr Shirk of the Gertrude and requested our captain to have him.

August 22

Dr Shirk came on board inviting me to make him a visit to his ship as he says a little change will do me good so captain gives me his gig and we go over to the *Gertrude* which lay a short distance [away]. I had a very pleasant visit Drs ship is a perfect little gem of a steamer. Such a complete little "man of war." Everyone on board had good quarters.

Dr of this steamer had been quite fortunate before he came on this monotonous blockade. His vessel captured a blockade runner and his share was near $10,000. Am told he ran through it while on a trip to New Orleans. The Gulf is getting quite rough so I took my leave of Dr who promises to come over and see me often. Wants me to join his steamer and makes me an offer to increase my pay from his own salary. Is an inducement should I leave the *Pocahontas*.

August 23

Last evening had much difficulty of getting on board of *Pocahontas*. Sailors lost several of their oars broken by hand pulling. However we succeeded and met no further mishaps. Today Dr Green[52] from the *Arizona* called.

---

different sets of words. Carlton R. Young, *Companion to the United Methodist Hymnal* (Nashville: Abingdon Press, 1993), 220, 793.

Dr. Shirk was Adam Shirk, Acting Assistant Surgeon. Callahan, *List of Officers,* NHC. Dodson will mention him again later in the journal.

52. There are several Greens who were surgeons listed in Callahan, *List of Officers*. The Navy Historical Center identifies the one assigned to the USS *Arizona* as S. S. Green, Acting Assistant Surgeon.

24

Mr Gould quite sick this morning. Several men on sick list today. After sick call made three dozen sassaprilla drops for Mr McCarter.[53] We had sent to New Orleans for the articles and I soon had quite a good substitute for sassaprilla soda water.

25

All going on well as can be expected. Captain promises to have a surgeon ordered here soon as possible. Today from the mast head comes word something is seen coming toward steamer. Proves to be a party escaping from the Confeds. Had them placed on steamer *Gertrude* to wait til the mail steamer came by to send them to New Orleans.

August 26th

Mail steamer came from the Rio Grande anchored sent the refugees and several paroled prisoners home. Some of the prisoners were from the *Harriet Lane* when she was captured.

27th

Very warm time on this coast. Seven men on sick list. Do the best can be done for them though I fully understand there should be more experience here. A smoke is seen. *Gertrude* is signaled to go to her. She proves to be lawful trader.

28

Early in the morning steamer *Arizona*[54] dipped her flag bid us

53. The reference to Mr. McCarter on this date and on October 2, 1864, is not clear. There is no McCarter listed in any of the sources previously cited. Dodson may mean Rodney Carter but he did not usually refer to his friend that formally.

54. USS *Arizona* was a 959-ton side wheel steamer, six guns. Originally called the *Carolina,* she was acquired by the Confederates only to be retaken.

good bye started for New Orleans. She had been our companion in the fleet this month and we miss her huge sides as they made us feel a little more secure having her with us.

Aug 29

Off Sabine Pass. What a scorching sun shines upon us. Orders have been given that as little work be done as possible. Close to mouth of Pass is the [iron] clad Confederate steamer *Sachem*.[55] We have only two steamers now guarding the Pass now that the *Arizona* is gone so we may look for an engagement at any time. At night a violent storm from the shore comes upon us and as the noise of its approach gave warning everything was made secure every precaution taken to meet the *Sachem* if she comes out. There are several other steamers with her and just such a night as this she may try to come out. The *Gertrude* is sent a little closer in shore and we are straining our eyes to see if a rocket goes up. Not much sleep tonight. How refreshing is the change of weather.

August 30 & 31

Off Sabine Pass. Expecting a surgeon to be ordered here any day. The health of the ship's company is good so I am not troubled much in that way. Nurse Randall has grown quite an important personage with the sailors. They seem to tease him on all occasions. He has had a long rest. He has had a bad finger which has prevented him from doing any hard work so is he detailed and rated nurse. I shall endeavor to let him have a good time as possible. So to protect him from the jests of the men I had him take up his quarters in the "sick bay" where he spends most of his time.

She was purchased from a Philadelphia prize court in 1863 and burned south of New Orleans in 1865. *OR*:II:1:38.

55. CSS *Sachem* was a 197-ton screw steamer, five guns. She was surrendered to the Confederates at Sabine Pass on September 8, 1863. *OR*:II:1:196.

The storm of yesterday prevented me from getting my bottling arrangements as they were all upset and disarranged during the blow. The *Sachem* did not venture out the night of the storm.

September 1, 2, 3, 4 1864

First of these days heavy blows. Old *Pocahontas* did pitch and roll. One, to look at one of "Lincoln's 90 days gunboats" as she lay a short distance from us, would suppose she would roll over or break her masts. Quite a contrast to the little Clyde built *Gertrude* that rides it out so gracefully. She is indeed a good sea boat and her officers say such weather is not uncomfortable to be on board.

Sept 5

Hauled fire. The Engineer Department to be fully inspected and gotten in order. Saw signal light which in a short time made out to be the USS *Penguin*.[56] The system of lights are quite perfect and each has a number in our navy and the arrangement of lanterns tells her number. For instance they are strung up say red, green, white would speak a number and any change of these colors would do the same.

Sept 6

Off Pass Sabine. The supply steamer *Admiral*[57] came up. Found a surgeon had been ordered to the *Pocahontas* and was on board the *Admiral*. We received quite a fine lot of stores provisions etc. Among other things that came were some fine Scotch ale and I thought I would sip a little for we had been without anything

56. USS *Penguin* was a 380-ton wood screw steamer, number of guns varies. OR:II:1:73

57. USS *Admiral*, a 1,240-ton screw steamer, five guns, was bought as a supply steamer and her name changed to *Fort Morgan* September 1, 1864. OR:II:1:28, 67. Curiously, Dodson's September 6 entry failed to note the name change. Knowing the ship, he probably did not even look at her name board.

good for so long. Thought it would not be amiss to try a little but I was not use to it and it made me quite "out of sorts" for the dull pain I had for several days afterwards over balanced all the pleasures of my appetite for it.

Sept 7, 1864

Off Sabine Pass. Today I am 22 years old but one will not have much heart to celebrate as I've done all yesterday for myself and this morning I feel quite out of spirits. Must brighten up a little as duties are before me. Was introduced to Dr Green who has been ordered to our ship. Have turned over all the official papers that come under his dept. He has had no experience and will have to get things a little in shape for him.[58]

Dr Shirk called in the afternoon. Wanted to know what I was going to do and again proposed to me if I left the *Pocahontas* to come to his steamer he assured me good quarters and offered me quite an increase in pay over what the government allowed me. Of course I cant leave the ship unless our Captain desires or gives his consent. The latter I have when I think I can better my condition.

Sept 8

Off Sabine Pass. Up to today Dr Green had only reported and not assumed any duty. I made my report and handed to him. There are two seamen who are totally unfit for the service and telling him that the sickness of Dr Mann had prevented them from being brought to notice so a survey was held and they were condemned. When the *Admiral* came up (supply ship) I took them with papers and had them sent to New Orleans hospital. Later in the evening met in Ward Room and had a

58. Dodson, who was apparently not a regular drinker, had a hangover on his birthday. The new doctor who joined the *Pocahontas* this day was Acting Assistant Surgeon Charles L. Green. NHC.

sort of business meeting of our choir. Dr Green joined us and took tenor part.

Sept 9th

U. States Steamer *Pocahontas* off Sabine Pass. From this date to the close of the month there was no special change in our life. Of course we had an occasional little event that would break up our quiet fleet but not a gun has been fired except in our practice. We have been quite vigilant as there are many rumors of an armed fleet up Sabine lake. On one day a very small craft was captured. She could not have been more than 30 tons. Came up a severe blow one night & her whereabouts was never known. We suppose she was driven to sea and floundered. Had a few men as prize crew.

On the 16th assisted Dr Green in amputating finger of one of the men. I gave him chloroform and all passed off well. During the month I have been performing duties of Dentist and a bottle of molasses will tell how much tooth ache we have had on board. Suppose salt provisions telling on them.[59]

One day this month the lookout reported "Sail ho." Soon loomed up in view one of the most unsightly of all crafts ever saw as the saying is. Someone must have built her himself and that someone had never seen a boat. She had steam on and was paddle wheel. As she moved along seemed in the turtle order as far as speed was. Well found her crew equally as queer looking. Her captain was called on board a true specimin of backwoods-man. He reported a sad tale.

He had fashioned this craft high up some river unbeknowns to Confeds and had run down and out to sea trusting his escape to some passing steamer. He wanted coal and provisions to enable him to reach the Rio Grande River. He was supplied and off

59. All the duties Dodson reports were typical for a Civil War hospital steward.

63

went the old barge. Later we heard he was a fraud for he attempted to run into Brazos River or some place lower on the coast and was wrecked. He wanted to set in and load some cotton.

October 1, 1864

Off Pass Sabine on board *USS Pocahontas*. We are knowing a pleasant time on board our ship. There is a much better living here than the warm days that we have been passing through. Was any chance for promotion and better pay that one could have a few more comforts I would not want a pleasanter place than the *Pocahontas* but by a new grade in the Navy she is rated lower than when we first sailed and my compensation is in like manner reduced as I am in this class of steamer 'tis rather unkind in a government that wants such places filled to require such qualifications as druggist and offers no better returns. I have been now here seven months and have thought as we may soon be ordered to New Orleans I would stay a little longer hoping by the time we come to port I could go home with a . . . of having stayed a respectible time. Seems I was unfortunate not to have resigned but I made a mistake and was too late. I should have gone as master's mate as that position would have offered a promotion.[60]

October 2nd

Off Sabine Pass. Everything moving along all right on board. Our sick list very short. Few are suffering from colds but not enough to give us much trouble. We are having it quite warm

60. In view of Dodson's understandable chagrin at the downgrading of the *Pocahontas'* rating and his own demotion as a result, it is strange that he declined Dr. Shirk's attractive offer to join his staff on the *Gertrude* (see entries for August 22 and September 7). Perhaps it was just a question of loyalty to the *Pocahontas* and her officers.

for so late in the season. Mr McCarter wanted me to spend the afternoon with him in the Engine Department. I was very fond of looking at the machinery and often during his watch would find way there. Used to be several 3rd assistants present and would have pleasant time.

One gained the name which we often gave him during one of my visits. He was describing to us the intricate machinery and when he explained himself about creating a vacuum he always called it *Wackum* so he was known to us by that name. 'Twas as much as we could stand to see *Wacuum*[61] trying to poise himself when called to muster. He and Barnes cut a laughable figure and I hardly know which had the advantage.

Oct 2nd *continued*

Off Pass Sabine. Just as the sun was getting quite low the steamer *Arkansas* came up from New Orleans with mails for the West Gulf Squadron also provisions. Received letters from Father and Mother. There has been a little stir among the officers and crew of the steamers in our fleet for on board the steamer there has been a case of yellow fever. It seems the man was taken few hours after leaving the passes of the Mississippi. The steamer is now at anchor and will sail tonight for the Rio Grande. The man died at 11 PM and the steamer then sailed away.

3rd

Sent in a picket boat. Came on a rough blow. She was driven out to sea and they had a rough time of it. The *Gertrude* was sent to look her up and when they found them they were much exhausted and tired and required stimulants upon their return.

61. "Wacuum" was Acting 3rd Assistant Engineer John H. Dougherty. NHC. In his entry for December 24, 1864, Dodson does identify "Wacuum" as "Doughty.

Oct 4 & 5

Off Pass Sabine. Dr Green is getting into the run of things and takes hold quite well. We are often together but not as was the case with Dr Mann. We keep a few on the sick list and now since the yellow fever was on the *Arkansas* every pain or change of feeling will occasion the greatest anxiety but we have a healthy crew. Our ship is kept well and every precaution has always been taken to keep their health good.

Our captain sent me a hymn and asked me to find appropriate tune so after a little change (for we are now about to eat our dinner) I will see how to please the captain. Will say for the captain he is very fond of wine and think he looks forward with pleasure for the Sabbeth to come so he can have us all on the Quarter Deck to take part in the exercises. He would make a good clergyman.

Oct 6th

Early in the morning found ourselves close to the brig receiving our coal from her til 11 o clock then we stood in for our station. The brig was sent loaded with coal for our fleet. Upon the forecastle of the *Pocahontas* sits a merry crowd Carter, Donell, Troyle Mr Donald and *Wacuum*.[62] They are singing telling jokes and getting the best of Barnes who can hardly keep from getting mad.

One day he came into the Dispensary and wanted me to make him hair dye. Well after he got it he used it too freely and though it changed his firey red whiskers it got on his cheek

---

62. The "merry crowd" on the forecastle cannot be completely identified. Carter, McDonald, and Dougherty all appear on the January 1, 1865, list of *Pocahontas* officers at the Navy Historical Center and on the April 1, 1864, officer's list at the National Archives. I could not identify Donnell or Troyle. There may have been personnel changes between October 6, 1864, and January 1, 1865, although Dodson mentions none.

and over his mouth so we come form an idea having such a figure head before us. What was the effect among such as are assembled upon the forecastle of the ship. The reason why we kept so long together today they were cleaning up ship and are ousted from our quarters.[63]

63. The page in the diary immediately following the entry of Oct 6 was left blank and on it later Dodson copied a song of David "My Father God in Whom I trusted." He paraphrased it into metre.

2.

U.S.S. ARKANSAS

Yellow Fever
OCTOBER 8, 1864 – NOVEMBER 2, 1864

Yellow fever was a deadly, incurable disease rampant in the South during the Civil War. Known as early as 1494, it derived its name from the jaundice-like color its victims developed. The following description is from an article in an 1881 naval encyclopedia based on numerous medical reports of the time.

Yellow Fever is "an acute, specific infectuous disease of a single paroxysm and remarkable malignancy." Found in tropical climes, it is limited to low altitude coastal areas, requires a humid atmosphere, temperatures over 72 degrees Fahrenheit, the presence of its specific cause and of decomposing organic matter. Shipboard personnel are particularly vulnerable.

It occurs after about a five-day incubation period and causes seizures and high temperatures. After one or two days the temperature moderates only to rise again. The patient then hemorrhages from the nose, gums, stomach (black vomit) and intestines (tarry stool), and the body assumes a yellow tint. Coma and death follow within a week. In mild cases recovery is slow.

Autopsy reveals fatty degeneration in the blood and liver which turns a brownish color. No medication is known to cure it and treatment consists of personal cleanliness, liquid diet, forced sweating and use of ice. The cause is unknown but is thought to be from a living organism or some substance generated by it.

Preventive measures include ship construction to minimize dry rot, ventilation, quarantine of ship and crew and strict sanitation as regards person, clothing, food and water. Chemical disinfection is ineffective, low temperatures cause it to disappear but does not prevent recurrence. Sulphurous acid gas at over 260 degrees Fahrenheit appears to kill all organisms and a naval board recommends its use to disinfect afflicted ships.*

The true cause, method of transmission, and treatment was not discovered until years later. During the Spanish-American War, yellow fever appeared among American troops in Cuba. Walter Reed, of the Army Medical Corps, a specialist in bacteriology and clinical microscopy, headed a commission to study the disease and proved that it was caused by the bite of mosquitoes infected with the disease, as Cuban doctor, Carlos Finlay, had earlier suggested. Doctor Reed believed that yellow fever was caused by a microorganism, and later research proved that microorganism to be a virus.

During the construction of the Panama Canal another army doctor, William Gorgas, devised methods of mosquito control that effectively eliminated yellow fever. Doctor Max Theiler, a South African researcher, developed a vaccine in 1937 that prevents the disease.

Compare the 1881 description of the disease with Dodson's undated addendum to the journal (pp. 143–44). The similarity is remarkable. It is not known if the addendum is contemporary with the journal or if he wrote it after he became a physician, although it was obviously written before the cause of the disease became known. It seems unlikely that he ever saw the encyclopedia article.

In October 1864, Admiral David G. Farragut reported to Secretary of the Navy Gideon Welles that "yellow fever has again broken out in New Orleans and a number of my vessels there, upon which it has appeared, have been sent to the Quarantine station. . . . Fifty cases have been reported from the hospital at New Orleans up to the present time, of which 12 have turned out fatally. We have had a norther for several days which I hope may have a benificial effect." This yellow fever epidemic had a dramatic effect on Surgeon's Steward Dodson, and is the subject of the next portion of his journal.

---

*Lewis Randolph Hamersly, ed., *A Naval Encyclopedia* (Philadelphia, 1881), 370–71; *OR*, I:21:679.

U.S.S. Arkansas

Off Pass Sabine. This morning the steamer *Arkansas* came up
from the Rio Grande river. She it will be remembered was here
on the second of this month and had the Yellow Fever on board.
Well there she lay flying the Yellow Flag as well as distress
signal. The disease has had nearly a week start and from description there is a melancholy spectacle on board. She seems to
be an object of terror as she rides at anchor pitching and rolling
for we had a very rough sea at this time. There is much signal-
ing between the steamers. Suppose they are trying to arrange
for her relief. Miserable and affected crew, little did I think that
in a few hours I should be with you to share the horror. For an
unvarnished tale would speak of scenes and sights that would
make us very sad to contemplate. I was sitting in Dispensary
and on looking up saw our captain. A very unusual thing for him
as we seldom ever saw him at that hour. Well in a short while he
called me Mr Dodson (heretofore naval rule had always given us
Sir).

He stated the matter freely using his own words. "Are you
aware what is transpiring on board the *Arkansas* and what an
unpleasant duty I shall have to perform unless someone will
offer service for that affected boat?" I for some time did not
suppose he had an idea that my services would be appreciated.
In speaking stated "were I surgeon of either of the vessels that
compound our fleet I should offer my services." Then he states
"Would you go if no one of my surgeons are willing" and yes
was given.

Now I cant say whether he further consulted surgeons Dr or
officers but in a short time he sent for me and finding he was
undecided I took the hint and said with much freedom Captain
if you desire me to go and think me competent to do the duty
only order me there and you will have no further trouble. I'll go.
Calling up Paymaster he asked me if I wanted my money. Telling

him no I would leave all things to his care and soon as my arrival at New Orleans would either come back or early communicate So after I had said good bye to friends [————] I came and said I was ready.

Now the difficulty was to get aboard the fever ship. She lay quarter mile or so from us but a high sea was running and we could not go along side without the greatest caution as would smash our boats. Well we soon had one of our largest cutters overboard and the swinging ladder was our place of departure as well as place of landing. Mr Chandler[1] [the] ensign took charge. We got off without incident fortunately. As we neared the *Arkansas* her ladder swings out from which hangs a rope guide. We are to row close to it and as we pass I have to make a jump and gain a footing that way. Mr Chandler commands "Care." Well you may suppose I took his counsel as far as possible. Well I gained the ship and when I reflect on it dont want to try it again. So much for that part of my journey.

Twas about 6 PM when I came on board. We immediately got underway. Could not help thinking of my undertaking and looking at the *Pocahontas* that was fast getting in the distance. She had been home for me for seven or eight months five of which I had not set my foot on shore and though there may have been some hours of lonleness within her "wooden walls" I had left some very dear friends and associations. Well but what a change from the healthy ship to this one. The full extent I am about to know before I go to sleep.

I find the *Arkansas* a large double deck screw propeller. She carries guns and is a mail supply steamer sailing from New Orleans and intermediate points far as the Rio Grande. Upon former occasions she has been a welcome visitor bringing much mail and fresh provisions to our fleet. I have had an interview

1. Mr. Chandler was later transferred to the USS *Kickapoo* with Captain Jones. See Dodson's entry for May 17, 1865.

with Captain Cate[2] her commander. As to his rank I dont know tonight for a common sorrow levels all. The best off here is the healthy and the strong. He tells me our hands are full. There are abundence of good quarters and he offers me his cabin very kindly. We are speaking of his officers who are below sick and upon the list I find her surgeon named.[3] This is indeed a bad state of affairs more than I had expected. Captain stated since leaving Rio Grande three have died and were thrown overboard. This was at 8 PM that the Captain and I finished our conversation.

I went to the Dr room found him in bed and from him learned enough. Paymaster Chief Engineer and many of the crew down with fever. The doctor was quite ill and though I did not want him to move would get up and with my support moved with me forward so as to give me a look at things and they were very bad. So many down some with stupor that nothing could arouse. Others are with nurses who are detailed to do all they can. Dr says "Do as you think best only let me get to my room." Poor fellow. He was quite disappointed as to his strength for the effort to go forward was too much.

What impelled me that night to visit every sick man I hardly know but I did see them all. I had a chance to see several cases while at Key West and had laid down in my memory many remedies and as one would suppose had read much of this disease under Dr Mann so was not at all ignorant as to the plans to follow. Seeing that many who had been ill a long time and in stupor would require no further trouble as they had but a short

2. Captain Cate of the *Arkansas* was Acting Lieutenant David Cate. He died while on duty on the Mississippi River May 4, 1865. Callahan, *List of Officers;* NHC.

3. Among those stricken with yellow fever were E. D. G. Smith, Acting Assistant Surgeon and Ed. G. Biship, Acting Assistant Paymaster. NHC. I could not identify the chief engineer who died of the disease.

time to live we made the balance as comfortable as possible. At midnight went to bed but for a long time lay awake as the steamer was rolling so violently.

At 2 AM she gave a heavy roll and out I came on the floor (I found the next morning many had been served the same). Was not long in gaining the deck. Who could sleep with such a night when I saw such a scene as would forget all of the affairs below decks. We had a perfect gale rigging parted and sails were blown away. Captain Cate says he never saw such a night or his ship behave so badly.

October 9

Wasn't we glad when the morning came. But for the light alone were we glad even if it did show us more plainly our misery and danger. Found several new cases. In fact there are so many that there is not enough left to keep up steam upon the vessel and our engineers are working very slowly. Conditions of sick deplorable. Most of them swing in hammocks and they are very uncomfortable at the rolls and pitches and in no way can they be made more comfortable til the storm goes down. This evening between 6 & 7 [two] men died. Buried them at midnight into the dark angry waves. Gloomy time.

Oct 10*th*

Aboard the steamer *Arkansas* on the Gulf. Today I had all hands to muster and come to the Dispensary window. Found a large portion much constipated so I thought to commence and give medicine as preventive. In our supply found a pound of Comp Cathartics Pills.[4] Each man that needed it has had a full dose. There is a large number of men aboard this steamer. Beside our

4. Compound cathartic, a mild laxative mixture of colocynth, extract of jalap, calomel, and gamhose. The compound could be given in smaller doses than would be effective if given individually. It was efficient and mild.

regular crew is a large number of refugees and exchanged prisoners. Most of them are on the spar deck. They are a rough set of
men. One of our officers tried to get the refugees to assist in the
fire department but found them unfit as well as unwilling. The
Paymaster has improved a little having arrested the vomiting
spells. Chief Engineer is a hopeless case. He has what is known as
black vomit and dont think he will last long. A light is reported.
Cheering news. South West pass is close.

Oct 11, 1864

On board steamer *Arkansas* off Quarantine. Came here this
morning. Ship reported to the Quarantine Surgeon. Up goes
our yellow flag and no more intercourse with the outside world
til we are adjudged free from the contageon. There are three
dead on board and in a short time that number will be largely
increased judging from the appearance of things below. Our
Chief Engineer has just died.

Had a talk with the Quarantine Dr and asked if it was not best
for me to return to the *Pocahontas*. As he expressed it I would
have to remain where I am because it would be dangerous to go
among the fleet and I would be wanted on board where I am. So
after examining my report and mode of treatment tells me to go
on. He would come off every morning. There are steamers and
vessels of all sorts with the green fever[5] in bound here. Close to me
lay the ram *Tennessee* her iron plating full of rough holes and dents
just as she came out of the Mobile fight.

Oct 12th

Off Quarantine. Dispatches from New Orleans. We are to stay

Colocynth is a type of plant; jallap is a powdered root; and calomel is mild
chloride of mercury.

5. Dodson's reference to green fever was probably meant to be yellow
fever.

here and all on board til further orders. Yesterday ice lemons and hospital stores came to us and I found them quite a blessing. Sent all the dead on shore and tis a frequent sight to see pine coffins going and coming over the ships side. There has been no new cases of fever today though there are several serious cases on hand. Many lying in stupor which will soon come to a fatal ending.

One case on board I have taken a special interest [in]. I found him for days totally neglected. He seemed to be a very consistent man and when I expressed my sympathy for his unfortunate neglect he calmly said how could he expect aid as so many others claimed our attention. He had no one with him to help and I must say he was acting the [————]. Found his trouble to be great inanition of stomach.[6] He had not taken food for a long time.

Everything I would give him would immediately come up. Lime water and milk sub mixtures of Bumister Oxzclate of Cennon all failed. Have tried small doses of Bromated Tincture of Iron[7] and have succeeded. Seeing the inanition abate a little. Later in the evening called to see him and found his nurse had continued to give him the doses I had directed and now he called for something to eat. Made a little beef tea and sent it to him. Midnight we sent another corpse ashore died five minutes ago. We dont keep them long on board.

October 13th 1864

Today warm. Captain sent to New Orleans for ice and beef. Had some oysters sent to us in the shell. Our surgeon has improved so much as to assist a little though he is confined to his room most of the time. Paymaster able to sit up. Most of the men look quite

---

6. Inanition means emptiness or wasting away.

7. No information found on bumister oxzclate of cennon. Perhaps it is an extreme misspelling. Bromated tincture of iron is a tonic (tincture means in alcohol solution) that raises the pulse and promotes secretions.

feeble. Use Quinine and whiskey[8] freely among them. Daily there arrive steamers here that have the fever on them and at time of writing we are quite a fleet at this place. Another dead man sent ashore tonight.

October 14

Off quarantine. Another death on board this morning. This was a rather pecular one. He had been in a stupor ever since I came on board. Could not get any medicine in him as his teeth were closed. So just this morning he was taken with Hemorrhages and when I saw him never saw such struggles. We could do nothing for him. He died very hard. In a few minutes he turned as yellow as an orange. We had a coffin on board. T'was not deep enough but we could not wait. *Things look desparate this morning.* He is placed in and, poor fellow, wish you had more room in your last prison. He is soon sent over to the shore where another shocking resting place awaits him. The lowlands of La will not admit of a dry grave so the coffin is often floating in [the] grave before it is finally covered. I find several of our men engaged making grave pieces to mark the spot of their comrades out of boards and lids of boxes.

October 15th

Off Quarantine. Received as hospital stores Beef, ice, medicines, etc. Have freely dispursed them the beef and ice as they will not keep long and thought turned to the [————] good to have such a change. So to-day all will fare well as far as eating goes.

Captain sent me a fine lot of oranges. How fine such fruit tastes when taken from their native place. Quite a difference from those we get up north.

---

8. Quinine and spirits is a mixture commonly used to treat and prevent malaria. Quinine is obtained from the South American cinchona tree.

In the afternoon although we had gone through such a life and still existed such an alarming disease among us we had a little life left among us. Several officers challenged all to follow them in a swim from mid ships to the bow of the boat against the current. So in shirt and drawers we go in. I shall never forget that effort and how near I came to being lost. Only for the kindness of one of the men who stuck to me and told me to keep close to the side of the steamer I reached the bow. Dont want to try it again.

October 16

Another man died this morning. Sometime before his death his coffin was commenced on board. So before he was cool he was placed in and hurried on shore. This is the sabbeth and most of it has past and just think of it. Still we are surrounded by such state of things as to make all forget anything but the misery we are surrounded [by].

17th Oct

Dr from Quarantine came aboard. Looking at the manner of our treatment expresses his satisfaction giving us a little advise. Still now from the appearance of things we will be here for some time. This is not very cheering. There is a company of young men in our mess who are very pleasant. We have good quarters in the Spar Deck. She is built with houses on this deck like an ocean steamer. My dispensary is a large room. Have a good berth in it and plenty of room. A Mr Anderson, one of the engineers of the ship, spends much leave time with me.[9] The Paymaster's clerk is [also] a very good friend of mine during these days.

9. Mr. Anderson was Acting 3rd Assistant Engineer George Anderson. NHC.

18th

Death of one more this morning. Sometime before he died his coffin was ordered. We have to hurry up things when they show that their end is near. We dont want them on board no longer than possible. I wrote the Flag Ship Postmaster at New Orleans for my letters. We are earnestly looking for a frost. This they say will be our only hope as it rids us from this disease.

19th

Our Executive Officer Mr Farrell commences to have the ship cleaned. Has pressed the refugees into service and some, with what is left of the ship's crew, are engaged in scrubbing, painting, etc. Others tarring rigging so in a short time things will present a more cheerful appearance. On this afternoon the refugees refused duty and are seen in groups. Trouble is expected but the officers on watch are all armed and ready.

20th

Off Quarantine. The weather is growing a little cooler. Mr Clemens our Engineer now in charge is taken sick, high fever.[10] Later in the day my old friend Anderson called and stated he had gotten ship's cutter and crew to row up the river a little. Wanted me to join. Was not slow in accepting. We went to the wreck of the *Verona* sunk by the Confederates. She was commanded by Capt Boyer.[11]

21st

Mr Clemens has had high fever up to 4 AM. Had given him CC

10. Mr. Clements was Acting 3rd Assistant Engineer. NHC.
11. USS *Verona* was a 1,300-ton screw steamer, ten guns, sunk in action below New Orleans April 24, 1862. *OR*:II:1:231. Acting Ensign Charles Boyer commanded her. Callahan, *List of Officers*.

Pills yesterday evening. Fever eases now he is sleeping a good thing.

22nd

Getting cool. Mr Clemens improving. CC Pills have had a good effect and I now give him Quinine as a tonic with spirits.

Oct 23, 1864

Off Quarantine aboard *USS Arkansas*. Sunday and sorry to say this has been badly kept by a boats crew that had with several others liberty to go ashore. They returned many had been fighting and most under the influence of liquor. Astonishing men so recently in the midst of such scenes as we have gone through should so soon forget themselves and do such things. If there ever was a place where a chaplin would have been in place it would have been with us for we have seen men perfectly rational dying then dead and buried and no word of cheer for them or Christian burial given their remains. During these times for recreation officers frequently have walks on deck and pleasant chats with them regarding their departments. The Dr, Paymaster, Mr Farrell, Mr Sculley, Mr Timken all of whom have shown me every mark of respect and kindness.[12]

Oct 24th

USS *Arkansas* Quarantine. Sick improving. Mr Clemens is much better giving him quinine beef tea etc. US steamer *NP Banks* lay a short distance from us. Yellow Fever on board. Think she just came from New Orleans. This evening the neglected man spoken of is doing first rate. Complains of no pain has no fever and increasing appetite. He is taking quinine and converses as if he

12. James Scully and Thomas E. Tinker were acting masters mates. NHC. I could not identify Mr. Farrell.

will soon be all right again. In the day time he swings in his cot on the lower deck and tonight I have left him comfortable requesting the Master at Arms to see that the large doors are closed tonight as a cool spell is feared would do him harm.

Oct 25th

Aboard *USS Arkansas* Quarantined on Mississippi River. Mr Clemens better. His was not an agrivated case and soon responded to treatment. Last night there seemed to be a little frost. I found it quite cool in the morning. Went to see sick. Found the man we had left so comfortable dead. The doors are very large of the steamer and he had been exposed to the draft all night. Had him soon on shore. Paymaster came up and found he had attack of Lichen External. Use of Glycerene and Aloes made him all well in a short time.[13] Mr Anderson again came for me to go boating. We go to the old *Verona* wreck, sail an hour or two up the river when we saw signal to return to steamer. Soon as we got safely on boat a storm of wind and rain came up.

Oct 27th

Off Quarantine. Am happy to say this morning our sick are nearly all comfortable and mending fast. Our ship by this time has been thoroughly cleaned and we begin to present a more healthy appearance.

Oct 28

Not any stirring event today. Mr Anderson called and finding me sleeping told the nurse to say to me "we dined at 4 PM." Our

13. "Lichen External" means a skin disease, but the term was used for more than one type of skin disease during the Civil War. Glycerine and aloes are soothing lotions we still employ today.

engagement consisted of a general meeting of all the mess where a report was served up. Quite satisfactory and the balance of the day we spent very pleasantly.

A German petty officer on board teaches me the Dutch land song to the tune of "Johnny Smokee." I cant twist my tongue or get the dutch language to call such a variety of musical instruments in their proper dutch or german names.

USS *Arkansas*

Off Quarantine. From the 29th to the end of the month we continued off Quarantine. There were no severe cases and maybe nothing that demands my stay here. Would gladly leave this place and gain a little liberty for we have been penned up here so long that it seems any change would be acceptable. During our spare time we frequently go short distances from the boat in small cutters. One day we went on board the ram *Tennessee*[14] a heavy iron clad that lay a short distance from us. One to see the iron plating would suppose no shot could do her any harm. Yet she presents a different story He sides are full of dents and front and rear so badly riddled as to almost look like a seive. She seems to have suffered most from the *Ossipee*[15] whose shot plowed through her open port often. It was damaged and would not close. This was in the terrible fighting that Farragut had at Mobile Bay.[16]

14. CSS *Tennessee* was a 1,273-ton wood screw steamer, a casemated ironclad, number of guns varied. She was captured on August 6, 1864, during the battle of Mobile Bay. *OR*:II:1:221.

15. USS *Ossipee* was a 1,240-ton wood screw steamer sloop, number of guns varied. *OR*:II:1:167. She was later commanded by Lieutenant Commander Meriwether P. Jones, former commander of the *Pocahontas*.

16. The Battle of Mobile Bay was one of the most celebrated naval engagements of the war. Admiral Farragut, with a large fleet, set out to destroy Confederate forces in Mobile Bay, Alabama, consisting of the ironclad ram, *Tennessee* and a number of wooden gunboats. In the ensuing

November 1, 1864

On board *Arkansas.* This month came in pleasant. The days are rather warm but nights are cool. We can sleep well though have to battle a little with insects that hum and sing around our pillow at night. Today sent letters to Clay and Uncle Ed.

November 2

We took a sail on the Mississippi in ship's cutter. Went to the levee and took a little walk inland resting under an orange grove. We had chance to enjoy some fine fruit. We are restricted in our distance to be within signal distances at all times. We return quite late in the afternoon. Found a letter from fleet surgeon Palmer[17] offering me same position on some steamer as Steward in Charge of Medical Department.

---

action the repeatedly rammed and shelled *Tennessee* was put out of action and surrendered. Admiral Farragut, aboard the flagship USS *Hartford,* was twice lashed in the rigging where he climbed to view the progress of the battle. When told of the sinking of the USS *Tecumseh* by a torpedo he reputedly shouted, "Damn the torpedos!" and ordered the fleet forward. Boatner, *Civil War Dictionary,* 558–59.

17. Fleet Surgeon Commodore Palmer was James C. Palmer, Surgeon October 27, 1841 and Medical Director March 3, 1871. It is not clear why Dodson referred to him differently in his entry of November 5, 1864. Callahan, *List of Officers.*

3.

U.S.S. HOLLYHOCK

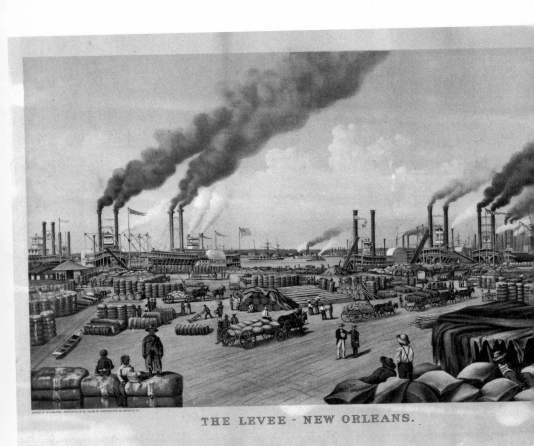

THE LEVEE - NEW ORLEANS.

Levee at New Orleans. (Courtesy of the Mariners' Museum, Newport News, Virginia

Destruction of the C.S.S. William H. Webb
November 3, 1864 – April 30, 1865

Quarantine Station
Mississippi River November 3rd 1864

The following order was placed in my hands today

Sir: You will proceed to New Orleans in the steamer *Ida*[1] and report to Commodore Palmer for further orders stating you have been for some weeks a volunteer assistant in the Medical Department of the steamer *Arkansas* by permission of the commander of the USS *Pochontas* to which steamer you belong signed D. Cate Act Vol Lieut Comd

The *Ida* is alongside and soon all is ready. Some twenty or thirty men are on board from our ship. Some will go to the hospital. Some are parties from the lower fleet and when they come on board their time has expired but had been guaranteed with us. We started. The *Ida* was a large tug boat. True she was armed but not much of a war craft.

Captain gave me his room or rather a bed in it and every thing went on pleasantly til I am called up at 1 AM. The convalescence under my charge to be delivered to the hospital sent for me and report that they are suffering much from cold. I find when gaining the deck that a chill wind is blowing and the poor fellows are all huddled under a few blankets or coats and not having any cover over them they are in a rather uncomfortable position.

---

1. USS *Ida* was a 104-ton steam tug, one gun. *OR*:II:1:106. She will be referred to often in future entries, and Dodson will unofficially act part-time as her medical officer.

Went up to the captain who is in the pilot house and talked the matter with him. He says he will remedy it in a few minutes as close to where we are he says is an old neglected cabin on shore so as soon as we round a little point of land we see it and are soon tied up to the river bank. The men go ashore and soon have a large fire built in the house. They are soon made quite comfortable for the balance of the night.

Nov 4th 1864

Arrival at New Orleans. Feeling badly went to a boarding house not far from the levee about three or 4 squares. Had a good dinner a refreshing nap then went up to Canal Street reported to Commodore Palmer. Received orders to report the following morning at 10.

Nov 5 1864

New Orleans. Received the following order

Sir: You will report on board the US Ship *Fear Not*[2] as Std in charge of Medical Department of that vessel. Signed P. S. Palmer Commodore

Immediately reported to Captain Hanson[3] commanding the *Fear Not* but found a young man had been ordered there in the same capacity that I am placed. Evidently there is some mistake but as my orders are from commodore my orders are respected by Captain Hanson and have taken charge of the Medical Department. I am quite aware that there is some mistake as two of us would never have been ordered here in the same position. Shall go up tomorrow and see Commodore Palmer.

2. USS *Fear Not* was a 1,012-ton wood sailing store ship, six guns. *OR*:II:1:83.

3. I was unable to identify Captain Hanson. He may have been John Hanson, Acting Master, who commanded the USS *Cayuga* as of January 1, 1865. NHC.

Nov 6th

A very stormy day so rough no boat left for shore so I spent the day on board. While here I take a look at the *Fear Not*. She is a full rigged ship quite large fine quarters moored between Algiers and New Orleans. She is a . . . sort of a supply and receiving ship no guns are aboard seems to be a place where convalescents are sent. Quite a large number are now on board. One I recognize as being on the *Pocahontas*. We sent him from the ship while at Sabine Pass. I am going to see if I cant get from this ship tomorrow.

November 7th 1864

Called to headquarters made my statement and was handed the following order "You will report to Acting Ensign J Elims[4] for duty on board the *Hollyhock* as Surgeon's Std in charge. Signed P. N. Palmer Commodore.

I will here state that there is a large number of steamers that either do not rate a surgeon or from scarcity of doctors can not be supplied so druggists are placed in charge. Their compensation is increased though as to grade officially they are only petty officers but are recognized as the Dr to the ship whose reports and orders for all necessary medical supplies of the vessel are always respected and filled. The above order will show why I went on board the *Hollyhock*. Feeling badly did not report until the 8th though Capt Elims endorsed my orders as having reported on the 7th.

On page 218 of the diary Dodson made the following entry:
Later
Paymaster J. E. Ryan at New Orleans had charge of several of the vessels accounts and it seems never transferred my name from the "Fear Not" a vessel

---

4. Captain Elims was Franklin Elims, Acting Ensign. Callahan, *List of Officers*.

I was only on two days. So my papers at Washington record discharged me from that vessel at close of war and not from Hollyhock.[5]

November 8th

Reported on board US Steamer *Hollyhock* and found her anchored off New Orleans. She is undergoing repairs. Painters are at work and machinists carpenters etc. A portion of her crew are on board balance on receiving ship. The Lieutenant of the steamer is from Baltimore.[6] Captain not being on board he read my orders and told me conditions of things and showed me my room and where the Dispensary would be found. A very few medicines on board and as there is such a mess of confusion while the repairs are going on will not order the medical stores until things grow a little settled.

November 9th

Noise and confusion too much for me and anyone knows who has experienced it what clammer is made during such times. Fortunately our room is a little remote from them and by staying in doors we are secure a little. Went on shore this afternoon. Met Dr Green and Emile Petor[7] from the *Arizona* which is in port.

November 10th

On board steamer *Hollyhock*. Spent most of day on board and

5. Dodson's official records at the National Archives do indeed show him as mustered out from the *Fear Not*.
6. The lieutenant from Baltimore was Acting Masters Mate Louis Milke (also listed in some records as Lewis Milk). Dodson identifies him by name in the addenda to his journal as does Callahan, *List of Officers* and NHC. Milke returned to Baltimore after the war where he must have met Dodson again, as both were members of the Maryland Naval Veterans Association.
7. Emile Petrie, surgeons steward on the USS *Arizona,* will become a good friend of Dodson's, and he is mentioned often in later entries. Dodson spells Petrie's name in a variety of ways.

while here will give a description of our little craft.[8] She is a side wheel steamer guns 3 compliment of men including Engineers and fire department forty. She has massive power for such a boat and has been used for various purposes. She sometimes carries dispatches, tows, docks vessels or any duty that may come suddenly upon her. She is supplied with powerful pumps independent of her regular motive power in case of fires among the fleet or on the levee. She has a clear deck (the lower one). Forward is the 40 lbs rifle gun aft the smaller ones. In the upper decks is captain's quarters aft of the wheel house. Further aft is a large saloon and on the sides are the berths four, one of which is my bunk. It is on the port side close to a window that commands a good view of the steamer's after deck. We call this saloon wardroom.

In our mess are the lieutenant, three assistant engineers, paymaster's clerk (or assistant) and myself five persons. We have a ship's cook and a steward to attend to us so everything on that line is well attended. Paymaster's clerk caters for us. We have good fare when in port for we can get just about what we please from the markets. While here today I found I had made a mistake leaving my clothes on the *Pocahontas* for it has been quite cool in the evenings and we are glad to get sometimes close to the cooks gallery.

I find the steamer has but two officers on board captain and the lieutenant and these are quite low grades. Captain is only ensign and the other master's mate. This is accounted for on account of the many vessels and scarcity of officers. The master's

---

8. USS *Hollyhock* was purchased March 5, 1863, by Admiral Farragut in New Orleans for $25,000 as a tender for ships of the West Gulf Blockading Squadron. She was a single-masted, 354-ton tug with double engines. She was sold at public auction in New Orleans on October 5, 1865, for $6,000. *OR*:II:1:102. There is a splendid and rare photograph of the *Hollyhock* in the Dodson papers.

mate is from Baltimore. Though rather a rough specimen learned that he is a very efficient man for the place.

November 11th 1864

Off New Orleans *USS Hollyhock*. 'Tis getting rather irksome to stay on board the steamer in an unfinished state. While the workmen, painters, etc are on board fixing up tis no use to try to keep comfortable. Our captain boards on shore. Have had a talk with him and til we can get a little fixed up will board on shore myself. Last night went to the theatre with Emile Petre a frenchman who is apothecary on the *USS Arizona* now in port. This ship was with us on the blockade off Pass Sabine.

Nov 12th

After breakfast we left the steamer and took a walk through the city. Went out the shell road and the lake. Find such beautiful little cottages out that section and real charming little spots close to the lake. At noon went to a boarding house and engaged a room. I was recommended there by police officer so after a little conversation with the lady of the house engaged board.

Nov 13th

Condition of things [bad] today. Captain says as there is such confusion on board and only a few crew if any get sick he would send for me. I need not come down for several days so as I feel a good rest is needed shall make myself content for a little while. After I get my room fixed up a little by the assistance of chambermaid and things have begun to look a little like home I began to think how much change I had gone through and I was indeed glad to rest. Had been suffering much from a fever which had been rather hard to ward off and get under control. Am taking large does of quinine and whiskey. Had to go to the marine hospital for printed forms tonight. There are several druggists at that place. Becoming acquainted spent several hours there.

Nov 14th

Thought best to report on board every morning so that nothing would appear that [I] was not doing my duty. Went down this morning. Am glad I did for one man was quite sick and thought best to keep him on board not to send him to the hospital as he seemed to have some dread of going there. Have him made as comfortable as possible.

My boarding house only five blocks away so left word, if wanted, to send for me. In the evening at boarding house parlor met several young men and ladies. Among the latter Miss Molly.[9] Had singing.

Nov 15th

Went on board our steamer. Had sick call. Found the case of yesterday improving. Another man reported himself as unfit for duty troubled with diarrheria. Administered oleum Ricini cum Tinct Oppi gtt XII[10] to be followed by other treatment tomorrow if necessary. Drew $30 from Paymaster's office today.

Nov 16th

Reported on board. Found the cases of yesterday improving. While here found the carpenters are working on the large saloon so I have them take a little order for my comfort. Have my birth fitted up a little better beside will want a few drawers etc fixed

9. Miss Molly, also referred to as Miss M, is mentioned frequently in later entries, sometimes at considerable length. For example see November 16 and December 8, 1864.

10. "Oleum Ricini cum Tinct oppi Gtt XII" means twelve drops of castor oil with tincture of opium.

up to add to convenience. In the afternoon generally feel a little feverish so make for my room on shore have a good sleep. Got up went down when the summons of supper bell rang and had a very satisfactory meal. Miss Maggie the daughter of our land lady came over to my chair and stated if pleasant "to come into the parlor during the evening" as a company of ladies would be there. I did so spent a pleasant time and as luck would have it the lady that I had previously met had to be escorted home. On offering my services was accepted. She lived quite remote and in no route of the cars so we had a long walk. After a space we arrived to her home a pretty little cottage seemingly to me on the outskirts of the city. Truly a very pretty place as viewed by the moon light this evening. She kindly asked me to rest awhile as our walk had been long but had previously learned her father was quite severe on all Yankees as he termed those who were in the U.S. Service. So thought best at time not to encounter the old gentleman but made arrangements to go to the theatre next evening with her.

Nov 17

Reported on steamer *Hollyhock*. Attended sick call. Work on steamer is progressing satisfactorily. Nothing further to do returned to boarding house study, writing, reading etc. At night went to the theatre as per arrangement

Nov 18

In the morning made my visit to the steamer finding all right in that direction [as] far as improvements concerned but found a man that had rather unpleasant symptoms. Soon packed him off to the hospital and in a few days he proved just as I had predicted a good case of small pox. Returned to my room reading on diseases we are liable to encounter here.

Nov 19

A rainy day. Reported to the steamer but everything is so "upside down" that did not linger there long. Returned to my quarters where spent the balance of the day. A Mr Bassett is boarding here. He is quite a musical character and a very agreeable fellow. He often comes in my room so we pass our time often quite pleasantly. He is quite full of fun and we are often endebted to him for an evening's enjoyment.

Nov 20

At New Orleans. Emile Petra called this morning and went to the steamer with me. We had a very good time on board in the saloon. He tells me he is going to accept a position in a drug store in the city as soon as his papers are processed from the ship granting him his discharge. In the afternoon per agreement went to the marine hospital to assist in dissecting a body that died of yellow fever. 'Twas very late in the season for the case and a little special interest was in it. The surgeons at the hospital gave us a good lecture for doing such a thing and took no stock in the actions of our youthful effort without their presence.

Nov 23

From this date to the close of the month the same duties in the morning went through leaving me the balance of the day at my disposal. Generally spent afternoon in study and reading. In the evening would occasionally make a trip to the theatre. Some days would enjoy a drive in the country. I had become acquainted with many of the ships crew then in port and picked up several good fees by treating some of them for such disease incident to their shore life.[11]

11. This probably refers to venereal disease. Gonorrhea and syphilis were common during the Civil War.

December 1, 1864

The *Hollyhock* is nearly finished. They have given her a complete overhauling so she will come out in no 1 order. My dispensary which is not a very large place is filled up. Best under the circumstances rather than to have the fumes of medicine and so close to our sleeping quarters had the side of a room on the gun deck filled with shelves etc for the medicines so will occupy it jointly with clerks the lieutenant of steamer and all of the ships writing will be done in the same room. As the medicines are all packed and ready at the hospital where we draw our supplies have ordered them to be sent down.

Dec 2nd

Today my clothes bedding etc came with letters from the *Pocahontas*. These were very acceptable as I had not heard for some time.

Dec 5th 1864

Left the boarding house as all was in good order on board. The captain said he thought best for all to come on board as we are expected to make a trial trip today. While here have concluded to live on board so entered ward room mess as before. Received crew or balance of them from the receiving or flag ship and steamed up the river on our trial. All works well.

Dec 6

Sent word to the house of my stay here. When I remain all day 'twas quite a change from my former life. The past months had been indeed quite lively but will soon get used to the change. Have good quarters here a pleasant saloon good bed and though I miss a little company still manage to get along very well.

Dec 7 1864

On board steamer *Hollyhock* at New Orleans. Our captain came on board took up his quarters. His wife came on to spend a few hours with him in his cabin. 'Tis quite cool and have a cheerful fire burning in our saloon today.

Dec 8

On board off New Orleans. I was sent on board the steamer *Ida* (a little tug carrying 20 men) to see a sick man. I had so often been there on the same duty til it was recognized as part of my employment to see to their crew's health. The captains of the *Hollyhock* and the *Ida* seem quite friendly and we are often alongside of one another so we look upon the *Ida* as a little of our company.

In the evening went on shore. Called to see parties at the boarding house. Found several ladies there among them Miss M and when she went home took the walk with her. When we came to her home thought if ever to avail myself of her invitation to come in 'twas time even if the old man frowns did keep up. He was opposed bitterly to having his daughter in company of the Yankees as he called us. Being a cold night buttoned up my overcoat so as to cover the buttons on my jacket and set out to enter. Found the house a pleasant picture to look upon. The parents sat in the midst of their children. A glowing cheerful fire was burning and shall never forget how inviting everything looked.

Was presented to the family and the father speaking of the cool spell (the never failing subject for beginners) quickened. Soon grew the heat of the room to such a degree as to make me feel very uncomfortable and his frequent invitations to draw my overcoat only added to my unpleasant feelings. I stood it out this time though I must admit it was a severe trial and was glad to feel the invigorating air on my way to the steamer that night when I got away from the fire which was never made to sit by in an overcoat.

Dec 9th

On board steamer *Hollyhock* off New Orleans. Emile Petrie the Frenchman came to see me. He is soon to leave the Navy and live at New Orleans. He has secured a position as druggist in a retail store.

Dec 10

On board steamer *Hollyhock*. The Thompsonian sweat[12] the old gentleman gave me in his parlor the night before last came near fixing me. On the way to the river the air was quite cold and so the change gave me a cold. Went to the *Ida* to see the sick man. Found him improving. Petrie called also Bassett so spent a little more pleasant time. Took a hot lemonade to break the cold.

Dec 11th

Went up this morning to the city. Called to the U.S. Sanitary Commission institution. Procured many articles of comfort for the sick department. This laudable enterprise seems to be much aided by women who secure donations from loyal people and give them out to the sailors and soldiers where in their judgment suggests. They gave me a silk quilt for my own use. Comes in first rate as most of my bedding was damaged en route from the *Pocahontas*.

Dec 12

Off New Orleans USS Steamer *Hollyhock*. Quite a commotion in our mess this morning. Two of our engineers are detached and

12. Dodson's reference to "Thompsonian sweats" is doubtless tongue-in-cheek. In the mid-nineteenth century "Thompsonian" referred to an offshoot of medical science that emphasized herbal or "home" remedies.

ordered to other vessels. This comes suddenly to them for they are quite comfortable and had made up their minds that they had gone into winter quarters on the old *Hollyhock*.

Dec 13

Off New Orleans. Today Mr. Boyce[13] (engineer) was ordered and came on board to fill the place of those who left yesterday. So we will have one less engineer than formerly. There are no serious cases of sickness. All the medicine that is required now with them is tonic. Steamer *Ida* sick are nearly well.

14th

Went on shore a little while. Saw Bassett for a short time then returned to the steamer. In a short time we went along side the *Arizona* and lay there a few hours. Saw Petrie and Dr Green. The latter came to the levee with us where we moored ship for the night. Had a cheerful fire in the saloon. Reading and study until 12 PM. Now I shall turn in for a good sleep.

15th

Spent the morning on board. After sick call (or rather after the hour as no sick are on the list for today) I took a trip to the city. Fell in with Mr Bowers. He was in charge of the Medical Dpt of the Ram *Tennessee* while we lay at Quarantine. He goes to Mobile this evening for orders. Just as I was going from Bowers who should I see but our Lieutenant. He was strutting along with an occasional lurch which he found much difficulty to contain. He saw me and 'twas amusing to see him trying to cross the pavements. He says he is going to have a good time tonight and from all appearances is in a fine way for it.

13. Mr. Boyce is Frank Boyce, Acting 3rd Assistant Engineer. Callahan, *List of Officers*.

When I returned to the steamer tonight. Found we had orders to go to the passes. Captain says will have to wait til the morning til the young man who is having such a good time turns up.

Dec 16th

On board US *Hollyhock* off New Orleans. She lay out in the stream. How and when did the young lieutenant come on board during the night we dont know but there was always one thing in his favor. He was always ready for duty on the morrow. A sound sleep would always fix him right so we are not now waiting for him but there is a dense fog and will start as soon as it clears up. Started and late in the night arrived at Pass a'Loutre.

Dec 17th

Steamed to Pilot Lain [or Lam].[14] Found a prize schooner that was going to New Orleans. Brought her to the head of the Pass. Then sailed to the south west Pass. Delivered orders. Found a brig there that had been captured some time ago with prize crew. We took her in tow came up to where we had left the schooner anchored. We then towed them up the river.

Dec 18th

On board *Hollyhock* on Mississippi River. Soon it got very foggy and were obliged to anchor off Quarantine. How well I remember this place where they had us cooped up so long in that fever ship. Tonight quite a lot of cotton was stolen from one of the prizes.

Dec 19th

Up anchors at 6 AM. Sun came out and we had beautiful day.

14. I was unable to identify the location of Pilot Lain (Lam). It is probably between New Orleans and the Gulf of Mexico according to the undated entry a short time after the *Webb* incident.

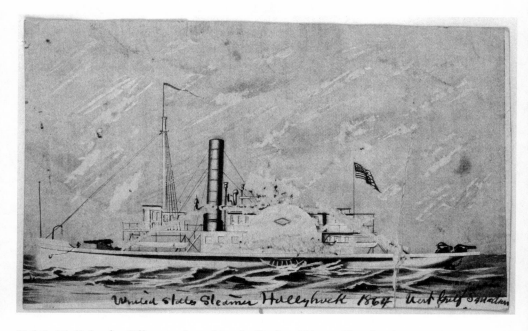

U.S.S. Hollyhock. *(Illustrated card in the Dodson Diary, Maryland Historical Society.)*

Made quite an imposing sight as our steamer is exerting herself towing these heavy laden vessels against a strong current. We move slowly along giving us a good view of the many plantations as we pass. At every one there seems to be quite a settlement. So many little outhouses and such a host of colored population. They seem to be out in full force airing and drying themselves. We anchored six miles below New Orleans tonight.

Dec 20th

Came up to the city. Continued on board until after tea when Mr Petry called and suggested a trip to the city. Having been on board several days was not slow in accepting.

Dec 21st

On board the *USS Hollyhock* off New Orleans. Very pleasant day. Some one gave me a little dog to keep on board. I had to accept as the man thought he was doing me a good favor. 'Twas a little beauty of a fellow and we used to derive much amusement from him.

The *Pocahontas* had come into port so started to see. Found her laying along the levee. You may know how friendly was our meeting. Even our sedate and dignified captain gave me a hearty welcome. He told me the first report they had was that I had died of the fever. This was previous to my writing for my things and Carter did seem very much pleased for as he said they had all debated on my sad misfortune when first news of my death came to them. So as long as the *Pocahontas* is here I shall have pleasant place to visit.[15] After greeting all my old friends found no important change had occurred. They are here for repairs. They have booked me for Christmas dinner which before leaving them have promised Carter to take with them.

Dec {23}

Spent off the city. Fine spell of weather. Ran a short distance down the river to the *USS "Onida."*[16] Delivered a lot of Texas reffuges and paroled prisoners.

Dec 24 1864

Off New Orleans. Sailed up the Mississippi River a short dis-

15. Dodson will spend much of his leisure time with officers of the *Pocahontas* after her arrival in New Orleans. Although contented on the *Hollyhock,* where he had made numerous friends, it is clear from subsequent journal entries that his heart is still with the *Pocahontas.*

16. USS *Oneida* was a 1,032-ton, wood, screw steamer sloop, ten guns. She was run down and sunk in Yokohama Bay, Japan, by the P&O steamer, *Bomba* on January 24, 1870. *OR*:II:1:165.

tance. Moved the *Selma* a dangerous drift of scows, coal barges etc as there was many adrift above the city. Sometimes they would strike a steamer and such [a] crash. 'Twas fearful to see the heavy coal barges as they moved after running into either a coming steamer or one at anchor plunge down. Then after the coal would tumble out they would leap up high into the air to return and be crushed into fragments by the flowing river. We got through this dangerous duty at noon. Returned to the city anchored.

Mr Carter and Doughty (Wackum) came aboard to see me. We had a very pleasant time rehearsing our life on board the old *Pochontas* at Sabine. We planned our day for tomorrow Christmas.

Christmas of 1864

After sick call on board took walk into city. Met Carter and several of our comrades according to agreement. Went on board the *Pocahontas*. Took dinner. Afterward went over to the *Hollyhock*. Found a general holiday there. The lieutenant was keeping it in good style.

After staying there til after tea went back to the boarding house. Took Carter and Doughty. We made several excursions into the city to see how things looked. A gay people are here and all enjoying themselves. Returning to the boarding house found quite a merry party had assembled in the parlor. Led by Mr Bassett they have a splendid time. Egg nog.

Dec 26th 1864

Lay off New Orleans. In the evening went to the city. Called to see the friends of last evening on board the *Pocahontas*. Well they are presentable though one or two are a little queer looking out of their eyes.

Dec 27

Ordered down the river with dispatches to a steamer below.

Somehow or other we are going quite swiftly and in a short time we run into a vessel. Did not do as much damage as one might suppose from the speed we were moving. Would have supposed the damage to have been much [greater]. However the carpenter soon had the *Hollyhock* bow fixed all right and we went on & delivered our dispatches. Returned to New Orleans late at night.

28th

Early in the morning started from New Orleans. Sent up the river. 'Tis a rainy spell and having no sickness did not go out of the saloon. A lazy life reading. Dont know where we have been this trip as the outdoors is so cheerless hardly even gave a glance out of the window. We have run considerable distance up the river but such things are of such everyday occurence and I dont believe they even keep a log unless we are outside so will have to ask captain when I see him all about this trip.

December 29

On board the *Hollyhock* sailing up the Mississippi River.

30

On board the *Hollyhock* down the Mississippi River.

31st

Spent all day on board. Arrived at New Orleans 5 PM in the evening. Went on shore. Found a message for me. If I came time enough to attend a sort of party. Did so. Had a pleasant time. By this time was prepared to meet the gentleman who refused so persistently to have any intercourse with the Yankees the first time I met his daughter. I was now on good terms with him and often found myself there. This evening went with his daughter from the party to his home.

U.S.S. Hollyhock

January 1865 [17]

This year commences with pleasant meeting and greetings of friends. Quite a number of officers from the *Pocahontas* called to see me. I have entered upon the duties of the year with full thanks. Through all the many changes of the past year I have been kept from harm. Not one harm has come to me for which I feel quite thankful.

A few days in the beginning of this month I have had very pleasant times. Nearly every evening finds me up town where I meet several officers of the *Pocahontas*. We sometimes take a trip into the suburbs of the city rather a cool place this time of year. After few evenings spent in manner described above I conclude to stay aboard. True I have not much company here but will be on hand if duty calls.

This month we had various duties. Sometimes we would be sent to the gulf. Sometimes up the river. Two or three days would be consumed on these trips. Twice during this month we landed the steamer at an orange plantation. That's what I would call it as saw more orange groves than anything. Our captain and lieutenant seemed to know this plantation from their previous visits.

Well we "tied up to the levee" as they call it. One night went to the planters home and a real jolly time we had. Planter captain and lieutenant got exceedingly jolly. I found in the daughters company more pleasure and kept myself all night. Left at 12 returned to the ship — a lovely trip (my friends had to remain at planters) and 'twas not easy to move to the steamer that dark hour so a good amount of difficulty presented.

When I arrived close to the steamer had to cross a sort of lagoon to get off the little boat that we came off in. Was no little job however succeeded. Got on board feeling sleepy and tired.

---

17. Beginning in January 1865, Dodson stopped making daily entries in his journal and continued it on a monthly basis.

When I awoke the sun was streaming in the window and we were steaming up the river.

Found beautiful flowers and some fine oranges in the saloon. The ladies had sent them by captain when he left the plantation. Bless those dear creatures. I have never seen them since but often will think of that adventure and the difficulty of regaining my steamer that dark night. The fruit was excellent being pulled the same morning they came on board. Their flavor was the best ever had since been in this section.

Well we came to New Orleans. On our way there came several little sloops with oranges for the city market. Our captain gave them a tow in exchange they gave us quite a lot of oranges. So upon my visit to see my friends shall give them some just taken from the trees.[18]

Went up during the month several times to see Mr H during the evenings when in port if I wanted. Went on shore and if chance would present would find myself in the section of the cottages. This was a pleasant section of the city where our lady friends resided.[19]

This month passed without any special event either startling or interesting. Same duties. Have lived on board this month and have everything pleasant though it seems that most of the evenings we now in port and 'tis quite lonely as the officers go on shore and leave me quite lonely.

We have a very sober sided engineer who stays on board it seems all the time and I may say always seems to stay in the same cloths. However he is reliable and quite a good piece of company even if several committees have waited on him to ask that he present at the table a more creditable appearance. Can always

18. It is surprising that the officers of a Union Navy vessel were so warmly received by the orange plantation owner and his family.

19. One suspects that the attraction at Mr. H's was Miss Molly rather than Mr. H himself.

count on his company but after conversation with captain think will board on shore this month.[20]

Later in the month Capt Elims was detached and B. Tarbell[21] special pilot appointed by Farragut to the *Hollyhock* in command. He commanded the *Ida* before and have met him several times so knowing the old gentleman think will be quite pleasant under him. His family are in New Orleans and when in port he goes up into the city at nights quite often.

New Orleans Feb 1865

This month the weather is quite cold and disagreeable so for the present am going to spend some time ashore. Went to the boarding house and engaged a room. The lady was very kind this time giving me a very nice room. In the morning go to the levee and little boat comes from the steamer. I stay there until about 3 PM up to which time if no orders come she is very apt to be there until the following morning. Sometimes we are sent over to Mobile Bay with dispatches, supplies etc. Tis rather risky sailing over there. So many torpedos are about that one never knows what time there may be an explosion. The *Ida* is over there now towing and different duties. She draws more water than we do (she being a propellor) and runs risk of striking one of these infernal machines.

There is a little small pox in the city.[22] On the 27th of this

---

20. Dodson does not identify the "sober sided" engineer of whom he gives a brief but revealing description. He mentions "sober sides" again in his entry of April 24, 1865. There were five engineers on the *Hollyhock* at this time.

21. Captain Elims, previously identified as Acting Ensign Franklin Elims in NHC, appears as J. Elims in Callahan, *List of Officers*. I cannot further identify Pilot B. Tarbell. He is listed as B. F. Tarbell, Special Pilot, in Dodson's Addenda and in the officers list of the *Hollyhock* at the National Archives.

22. Smallpox is an acute, eruptive, contagious disease caused by a virus

month was taken "Robert Kay."[23] The men up to this date had been unusually well. Total number on the sick report for the first quarter only showed four persons had been on the sick list in all. This with an average number of ships company 40 was a miniscule percent. This case awakened a good amount of interest. Was not long in turning him over to the mercies of the hospital at New Orleans and now little steamer is free again. 'Twould have been a blow to our enjoyment had the disease developed itself among the crew but was happy to see we had no fresh cases.

How cold it is here. Fires on board will hardly keep us comfortable. This month I find boarding with us at the boarding house on shore the following officers of our navy. As are all old friends of mine that have been introduced by me the landlady gives me good attention. Room well attended and fired up for me every afternoon. Dr Green USS *Pocahontas,* Dr Green *USS Arizona,* Rodney Carter *engineer USS Pocahontas,* John Doughty engineer *USS Pocahontas,* Ben Tucker master mate *USS Pocahontas,* Charles Sidney, Mr Caswell Winters steamer *Estrella* and Bassett our musical friend.[24]

I forgot Barnes. Last but not least he figures here. When I presented him took the precaution to request that he put in his good behavior and no "shenanigans." Says he would have no objection at getting acquainted with some ladies but the young man has a wife and we have the best of him. Barnes has not changed much neither has his "lean and lank" sides expanded much since he has been on the blockade. Carter calls him "Barnzy" and will always give him a joke whenever chance presents. He's a character you often read about but never meet.

---

and marked by the onset of chills, high fever, backache, and headache. Skin eruptions appear in two to five days.

23. Robert Kay appears to be an enlisted man. Dodson usually identified only officers by name, with a few exceptions.

24. The officers living at the same boarding house with Dodson have

When there are so many young men we manage to have a good time. My room is quite a meeting place and sometimes have to call them to order. When a certain one comes in he will insist on living over old times and having a good time generally. The landlady gives us a room where we can all assemble. This arrangement relieves me very much. So the chewers and smokers can have their full benefit.

One night we had a large fire among the shipping. Our steamer was called into use to save property. Her large marine pump worked handsomely doing good service. Fire extended to the cotton, hay etc on wharf. Several steamers consumed.

One evening this month made a call to see a lady friend.[25] Found her sister in an adjoining room making quite an effort to sit up and playfully asked if I wanted to see a sick person. Her father and mother seemed rather uneasy in her account. She has been complaining several days and now has much pain in back. Had a very disordered stomach a few days ago.

She is a young lady about 16 years and up to present time quite healthy. She was exceedingly stout and good natured. Suggested that their family physician be called in the event of her not getting better. Suggested a dose of Sal Rechell.[26] Next went, which was two days, to see Mr H. Found the daughter still in bed feeling badly. Asked if I would see her.

Here was an unenviable position but as Mr H insisted went to see her. Soon it occured to me she may have the "small pox" and made known the opinion to the family who were very much distressed but did not seem to mind the disease as much as they did the isolation it would bring to the family.

---

been previously identified. The *Estrella* officers he names are Acting Masters Mates Charles Sidney and E. G. Caswell and Acting 3rd Assistant Engineer James F. Winters. He garbles their names in his entry. NHC.

25. The unnamed woman friend in the Miss H smallpox account is Miss Molly, the patient's older sister.

26. "Sal Rechell" probably refers to Rochelle salts, which was potassium

I advised them to send for their physician but they seemed to be entirely at loss what to do. Telling them the scare may be premature wait til the morning giving her a little warm drinks during the night. Next evening called was surprised that no physician was called. Saw there was no mistaking it this time.

The father and mother seemed very sad and was so much worried about younger children and its getting out. Suggested that the disease was only to be nursed properly. They had a play house quite remote from the cottage so proposed that the young lady be placed there. Her mother gave her attention and kept [her] away from balance of family as much as possible. So we prepared to carry this out quietly and have given word to call and see her occasionally.

Ordered small doses of cream of tartar. She was much afraid of being marked. Made her a mask when the pustules were healing. Spread dilute Hzdrany Ointment[27] on them. She was quite obedient did not scratch herself and when she came out was all right. Last I saw of her was her original self. This was quite an adventure and had a very pleasant ending for at all times I was welcome to Mr H's home.

Later part of the month very cold ice formed on the levee. One night this month we had a stag party at the home. I was sorry Vacuum came drunk. Had him put to bed. Bassett playing music. Carter singing with Dr Green. Barnes (the Yankee) room is close and we hear Paymaster Wright there making a stump speech. All the response from Barnes is a grunt.

March 1865

Our captain seems to think all that is necessary for me to do is to

---

sodium tartrate and was used as a carthartic. Cathartics induce an emptying of the bowels.

27. "Cream of tartar" is potassium bitartrate, also a cathartic. Cathartics were often given to smallpox patients. "Hzdrany Ointment" is probably

continue reporting every morning there in case we are wanted on any trip will give me notice. This plan may work well for a short time but our trips may be extended as to place me in an embarassing position so have arranged to keep my room and when away on steamer deduction will be made for board etc. This life ½ on shore and ½ aboard calls for extras so manage to occasionally make an extra five or ten whenever a chance presents.

This month William Barton, Lieutenant of the *Lackawana*[28] called to see me bringing word from Bro Rich. He had promised him to find me out and see how I was getting along. The *Lackawana* is in port now and her captain Emmons[29] is the ranking captain of the port or in other words was the flagship. During this month we made frequent trips to the Gulf and to Mobile Bay. The little steamer *Ida* was blown up by a torpedo there. Several of her men killed.

On return from one of the Gulf trips once this month I went up into the city for a little change and had permission from captain to report at 10 next morning. Went up into boarding house and passed the night. When I arrived on the wharf found the *Hollyhock* had been ordered away suddenly to the Gulf. I went for several days to the wharf and made inquiries from the fleet in port but no tidings from the boat. Now thought here was a nice thing perhaps the very time one is needed to have been away was rather a serious thing to contemplate.

Stood it for four or five days then called to headquarters to report the case to Commodore Palmer asking for information regarding the steamer and requesting to be sent to her. Nothing can be heard this morning from the *Hollyhock*. Received order to

---

Hydrargyri unguent, a mercury ointment used externally to prevent smallpox scars.

28. USS *Lackawanna* was a 1,533-ton wood screw steamer sloop of war brigantine, fourteen guns. *OR:*II:1:123.

29. Captain Emmons of the *Lackawanna* was George F. Emmons,

report on board the *Portsmouth*.[30] This vessel lay off New Orleans as sort of receiving ship. When I arrived on board supposed there would be no detention but found had to stay on board that night as well as the succeeding day and night. On the second morning was called up and informed the *Hollyhock* was approaching. A boat was lowered and I was soon on board in my old quarters and real glad to find the old steamer above water and no disaster had attended her.

The captain says when he was ordered to Mobile was quite early and supposed I was on board forgetting I had gone ashore. When far down the river discovered my absence but thought best to proceed as the orders were hastily given. Sailing along the coast she struck a reef or mud lump and remained there two days. Fortunately the gulf was moderate most of the time and she sustained no injury. We had given her up as lost and her arrival was to me quite a relief.

Captain says twas his fault that he did not notify me as I was only four squares off. Why I was kept on the receiving ship seems to have been that I had been ordered there til *Hollyhock* came in port and as my papers did not specify why I was absent they would have inferred that my place was with them til her arrival.[31]

April 1, 1865 [32]

On board USS *Hollyhock* off New Orleans. From the experience of last month I shall always try to be within signal distance of our steamer so have taken up quarters on board again. Our work first part of this month consisted of constant towing and docking

---

midshipman 1828, captain 1863, retired as rear admiral in 1873. Callahan, *List of Officers*.

30. USS *Portsmouth* was a 1,022-ton wood sailing ship sloop of war, number of guns varied. *OR*:II:1:182.

31. Technically Dodson was absent without leave.

32. Although dated April 1 the entries actually extend to April 24 without further dating.

vessels. In fact we are now considered an effective tow boat. We generally tied up to the levee but the men seemed to want such an amount of liberty on shore that we now anchor out in the stream.

We are always under steam or what is called banked fires ready for any duty at shortest notice. All that is necessary in the engineers department is to spread fires and steam will soon be up. Went up this month to marine hospital and selected quite an assortment of medical supplies for the steamer.

Have good chance to visit in the city so often during this month go up to see Mr H family. His eldest daughter now seems like an old friend and Maggie[33] her sister seems to always have something good in store for me. Says she shall now forget that "false face" I made her put on when there was danger of her good looks being in jepordy. They are a very happy family and shall often think of their kindness and many pleasant times I spent with them.

Our Lieutenant went north this month. This leaves us so far with no line officer except captain who expects a relief soon. Mr Bassett comes on board to see how things are "improving" as he calls it. We miss Lieutenant Franks on board. He lives in Baltimore and is a wild specimen though when on duty was an efficient person.[34]

I have missed the officers of the *Pochontas*. She is now on the Gulf of Mexico doing blockade duty. Learn some of the officers are ordered to other steamers. Think Carter has been sent to the

33. The ailing sister was Miss Maggie H. Miss Molly was the eldest daughter of the family.

34. The reference to Lieutenant Franks is puzzling, for earlier Dodson has identified the Baltimore lieutenant as Louis Milke.

A mate named William G. Franks was cited for gallant conduct at Yazoo City in 1862, but Milke is listed among the *Hollyhock's* officers on January 1, 1865. NHC. On April 24, Dodson again mentioned the departure of Lieutenant Milke and noted that no replacement had arrived.

Estrella and Captain M. P. Jones has gone to one of the monitors in Mobile Bay. I think her name is the *Kickapo*.[35]

(next three lines are badly faded and illegible}

They have quite a fleet over there and often I have seen them loom up in the distance. They should have done something effective and startling.

One of the most pleasant sail ever had was on a Sabbath of this month. Coming from the passes of the Mississippi River a beautiful day. We ran in close to the banks as to almost be able to jump on dry land. The shore was lined with people and when close to the city late in the afternoon the banks were crowded with Ladies & Escorts. A beautiful picture.

35. USS *Kickapoo* was an ironclad steamer with two Ericsson turrets and four to six guns. *OR*:II:1:121.

In Pursuit of the William H. Webb

Beginning with his entry for April 24, 1865, Dodson describes another memorable Civil War experience, the encounter of the Hollyhock *with the Confederate ram* William H. Webb. *It is probably the only surviving personal account of the final stages of that event. The following narrative serves as a prologue to this portion of his journal.*

In April 1865 there occurred one of the most daring naval exploits of the war. The CSS Webb *left its haven in the Red River and descended the Mississippi River in an attempt to reach the open sea and operate as a commerce raider. She traveled almost 300 miles, passed through four naval districts, tricked or outran a score of Federal ships, and successfully passed the fleet in New Orleans, all without firing a shot. About twenty-five miles south of the city, almost within reach of her goal, the* Webb's *venture ended in failure.*

The description of this incident occupies about twenty-five pages in the Official Records, *most of which cover the earlier phases with no detail on the end. The New Orleans newspapers gave it wide coverage. The* Times-Picayune, *for example, issued an extra the day after it happened and published numerous articles on subsequent days.* Harpers Weekly, *a widely read national journal, published an article and a dramatic artist's sketch.*

The William H. Webb *was a 655-ton steamer with double walking beam engines, extremely fast and powerful. Built at New York in 1858, she was owned by the Southern Steamship Company and was well known as a tow boat in New Orleans. In 1861 she was issued a privateer's license but was never used in that capacity. In early 1862 she was confiscated by the Confederate army and converted into a ram for operation on the Red and Mississippi Rivers.*

A ram, as the name implies, was a vessel with a reinforced bow for sinking or disabling other ships by collision. Some had armored casements to cover the guns and sloping sides that caused shots to bounce off. Others were protected by

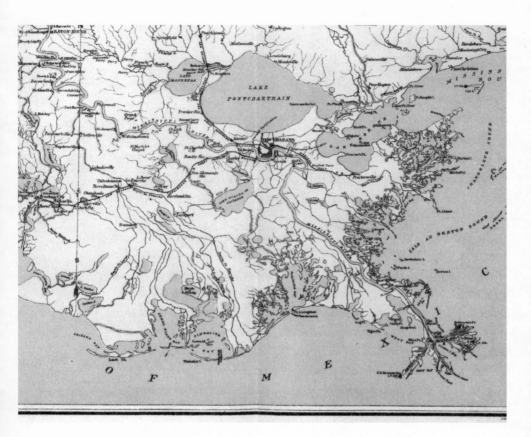

The Mississippi Delta, where the William H. Webb *attempted to break out to the Gulf.* (Official Records of the Union and Confederate Navies in the War of the Rebellion, *I:18:131.*)

cotton bales. The Webb *was of the latter type. Under army command she participated in the sinking of the USS* Indianola *in February 1863. In early 1865 the* Webb *was transferred to the navy for duty against northern commerce.*

Her commander was a twenty-four-year-old Mississippian, Lieutenant Charles Reed, a graduate of the United States Naval Academy who cast his lot with the South. Especially selected for this venture, he had prepared well. Under his direction the Webb *was armed with three guns and five hundred-*

pound torpedos, one of which was fastened by extending out over the bow. Only one day's supply of coal being available, she was loaded with wood for fuel and cotton bales for protection and eventual sale if her attempt was successful. Her crew numbered forty-five. Depending on timing, surprise, and speed to get him past the Federal ships, Reed planned to disrupt communications along the way and leave the Red River at night.

About 8.45 P.M. on April 23, 1865, the monitor USS Manhattan, *stationed off the mouth of the Red River, first noticed heavy smoke, then a small vessel without lights emerged from the river traveling very fast. When she refused to acknowledge the* Manhattan's *challenge the monitor fired two shots at her as she passed without visible effect and sent up rockets to warn ships downriver. A newspaper correspondent aboard the USS* Saratoga *said that the* Webb *nearly hit her as she headed south at a high rate of speed and that the* Saratoga *had to back up to avoid a collision. The two ships were less than fifteen feet apart as the* Webb *passed.*

The USS Lafayette, *USS* Vindicator, *and USS* Lexington *started in pursuit and the first two followed the* Webb *as far south as Bayou Sara, forty miles below the Red River, before giving up the chase. Others who joined the pursuit were the USS* Ouachita, *USS* Fort Hindman, *and USS* General Price. *None came close to catching up with the* Webb.

According to plan Lieutenant Reed stopped several times to cut telegraph wires, thus preventing ships down river from being alerted. The fast moving Webb *passed other vessels before they realized what was afoot and arrived about ten miles north of New Orleans at about noon on April 24. Here she ran up the American flag at half mast in recognition of the assassination of President Lincoln. She was, up to this point, undamaged.*

But word of her coming had finally reached the city and Forts Jackson and Saint Phillip to the south guarding the entrance to the river. Ships of Admiral Farragut's West Gulf Blockading Squadron at New Orleans were ready for her for what little good it did them. Four ships, the USS Lackawanna, *USS* Ossipee, *USS* Pembina, *and USS* Port Royal *opened fire on her. Reed lowered the American flag and raised the Confederate banner in its place.*

There is confusion in the Federal reports as to how many times the Webb *was hit and by whom. According to several prisoners from her crew, she was struck three times. The first entered the bow just above the water line, dislocating the torpedo, which had to be cut loose. The second grazed the smokestack and wounded one man, and the third hit a cotton bale. Not seriously hurt, she continued down river at full speed, dipping her flag in mock salute as she went. The greatest damage inflicted by the fleet at New Orleans was done by the Port Royal, whose shells struck several houses in the city. An examining board assessed the damages at $200. The Navy refused payment.*

The Hollyhock and the Florida were dispatched in pursuit, the Hollyhock, as swift as the Webb, far in advance. The Florida would not reach the scene until the action was over. At McCall's Point, some twenty-five miles below New orleans, the voyage of the Webb ended. The mighty USS Richmond, 2,700 tons and twenty-two guns, inbound from Mobile Bay, was anchored repairing her engines. At 2 PM, seeing the Webb approach, she fired three times but did not hit the ram. Unaware that the Richmond could not pursue him, Reed ran, the Webb aground and set her afire. The crew abandoned ship and sought to escape inland.

Neither Reeed nor the the captain of the Hollyhock filed reports after the action, but the accounts of three members of the Webb's crew, who were captured and later questioned by the famous detective, Alan Pinkerton, described her final moments. Lieutenant Reed was timing his passage to pass Forts Jackson and Saint Phillip at night. On encountering the Richmond, he considered turning back to engage the sole pursuing gunboat, the Hollyhock, which was about the same size and armor as his ship, but, fearing the Richmond, decided to destroy his ship rather than let it fall into enemy hands. This account agrees closely with Dodson's journal regarding the Webb's final moments.[36]

36. *OR*:I:141–70, passim; *Dictionary of American Naval Fighting Ships*, 2:581; *New-Orleans Times Picayune*, April 25–26, 1865; *Harper's Weekly*, May 20, 1865; Callahan, *List of Officers.*

1865 New Orleans {April 24, 1865}

On April 24th we lay at the wharf at New Orleans. I was in my Dispensary, the captain was with me. I had been doing some writing for him. He looks up and gave me a sudden start and he ran to the window explaining "Now we will have a time of it." Bang bang went cannons from the fleet. As I looked up I saw a steamer. She seemed to be almost flying by us. Our captain knew her well and says "tis the ram Webb." She had run out of the Red River, passed Porter's fleet cutting the telegraph wires. Her passing New Orleans was very sudden though some information was at headquarters and only a few minutes difference knowledge was known [on] the *Lackawanna*. Sufficient for Mr. Burton to have a few guns ready which they gave her as she passed. She had her torpedo arrangement and tried to blow up the *Fear Not* who was watching her.

{*Later note in different ink*} This boat a ram was quite formidable and was mentioned by General Grant in his *Memoirs*, 1st volume page 465 Seige of Vicksburg.[37]

She was going so fast when she made the turn that it broke and the old powder ship was saved. The rebel craft was flying the stars and stripes at half mast to deceive us (our fleet had them so on account of Lincoln's death) and kept it so til she passed the fleet then she raised the Confederate flag. All this done in a few minutes. Several shots struck her hull and some struck the cotton bails which made the crew scatter some when seated on top of the cotton but when one of the *Lackawanna*'s shots crashed into them they soon left the exposed places.

37. General Grant records how the *Webb*, with several other vessels, pursued the USS *Indianola* on the Mississippi River north of the Red River. The *Indianola* battled the Confederates for an hour and a half, during which the *Webb* and others rammed her seven or eight times, mortally wounding her. The *Indianola*'s armament was thrown overboard, the ship was grounded and her officers and crew surrendered on February 24, 1863. *Personal Memoirs of U.S. Grant*, 2 vols. (New York, 1885), 1:465.

Captain Emmons Seignor Captain was in command at this time at New Orleans (Capt of the *Lackawanna*). He sent Lieutenant Commander Ghehardi[38] to our steamer with instructions to try to run her down or press her to the forts below. We have banked our fires and started immediately for her. She had a start of ten minutes and full head of steam. We started at 12.40 PM, all stir and confusion aboard. Steam is fast going up and in a few minutes the old *Hollyhock* will be doing her best. Tis a beautiful sight to see this race. The ram is fast and from the dense volume of smoke she gives forth everything of inflammible nature to make steam is being consumed.

Our Chief Engineer Mr. Wilcox[39] seems to be in his element for using his expression whenever he was elated he says "man oh man look at our steam guage." A full head is on her and we have commenced the race in earnest but the *Webb* holds her own. She is fast and has the start and for some time cant see any difference. Our forward rifle gun opens on her first at random to attract the fort's notice but soon a more direct aim is taken. Lt. Gerardi [Bancroft Gherardi added later in different ink] is on the foward deck with the gunner and seemingly has command. Tis good that he is there as this race has happened at a bad time for the *Hollyhock.* Not one line officer except our captain. Our Lieutenant Mr. Milke had left a few days ago and no one had come to fill his place. Dont I wish that he had been here (Mr Milke). I think a

---

38. Lieutenant Commander Bancroft Gherardi, midshipman 1846, Lieutenant Commander 1860, retired as a rear admiral. At the time of this affair he commanded the *Port Royal,* an 805-ton side wheel steamer, ten guns. The *Port Royal* was the ship that damaged houses in the city while firing on the *Webb.* Gherardi was a member of the board assessing the damage. *OR*:I:22:xv, 729, 165. Callahan, *List of Officers.*

39. Alex Wilcox was Abraham H. Wilcox, Acting 1st Assistant Engineer. Callahan, *List of Officers.* Dodson apparently confused his first name with that of Alexander McDonald, Chief Engineer of the *Pocahontas,* when he referred to Wilcox in the addenda.

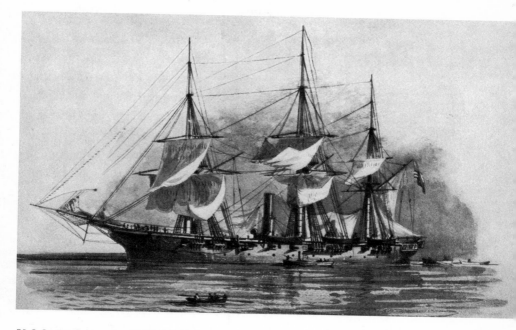

U.S.S. Richmond. *(Official Records of the Union and Confederate Navies in the War of the Rebellion, I:18:frontispiece.)*

different result would have been. Such was the condition of things on board in the face of an enemy of superior strength.

We were making toward him and the key to the chest containing muskets sabers pistols etc cant be found. Our Captain is at the Wheel. Chief Engineer on watch with 2 assistants leaving one sober sided 3rd assistant off watch with nothing to do below who comes up to the upper deck. We force the arms chest open give to all idlers on the upper deck a gun which we loaded ourselves and hand to them. We hurry to protect Captain as he is much exposed. This may appear a strange proceedings but the case demanded it. Gherardi was on the lower deck. Our Captain had much to do at the wheel and no one was left to guard the upper deck.

We are now doing our best but it seems little gain is made upon the *Webb*. We can see the men plainly and observe their movements for the past 20 minutes we have [been] continually on her. In the distance we see the tall spars of a steamer looming up. (proved to be the *USS Richmond*). About this time the *Webb* turned and headed for us and we now thought the "tug of war ad come." Will say for our captain he told the engineer to open wide the throttle valve and give her all the steam possible. Standing at the wheel firmly he aimed the *Hollyhock* to meet the coming ram. We are now so close that [we] expect shock any moment. They are firing quite rapidly with the forward gun.

Suddenly hear a shout. The ram has run into the bank and quicker than I can tell we are upon them. She careens and most of her crew go over the bows and fly into the woods. We soon find the ram on fire and some of the captured men say "magazines are trained to blow her up." Our pumps are soon at work. Our *sober side* engineer runs on board and lets off the safety valve and what a head of steam. No wonder she went so fast. I am soon with *sober sides* on the deck and there is some excitement. The hose is playing on the fire. Gherardi takes a sudden alarm and orders our vessel to back away as he says "We will all be blown up" so we are backed off.

As we are some distance from the ram we see several of our sailors on her deck. Gherardi cries out "Jump overboard and swim or you will be blown up." I was struck at the coolness of the seamen. They quietly lowered the cutter from the burning vessel came bringing two or 3 of the captured crew found entirely overcome in the fire room. They came aboard just as found and would say they had a very haggard experience.

Our sailors who had this little trip on the burning ram seem to have been very much composed and had we had our lieutenant think such composure as they exhibited led by him would have saved us the craft and perhaps given us a good sum of prize

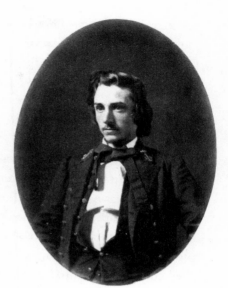

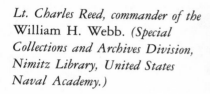

Lt. Charles Reed, commander of the William H. Webb. *(Special Collections and Archives Division, Nimitz Library, United States Naval Academy.)*

money. She was full of cotton and soon down the stream could be seen rolling from her decks.

One little incident connected with this exciting episode would have been quite a satisfaction in the end if Gherardi had not obtained the article I had desired to preserve as a remembrance[40] of this affair. As we lay alongside of the burning craft her flag was only a few feet from the deck and as we were about to back off from her I saw it and got Willie, our stewart, to jump across and get it. He gave it to me and I placed it under the head of my bed or rather I had Willie do it.

In an hour or so quite a large fleet came down from New Orleans. Some were heavy vessels and did look quite formidable coming down under full head of steam. They had gotten upstream and in the case of the ram getting past the forts to chase

40. I was unable to determine the current whereabouts of the *Webb*'s flag that Gherardi took from Dodson. It is not listed in M. Michael Madaus, *Rebel Flags Afloat* (Flag Research Center, 1986).

her to sea. When they found her burning and our short lay off looking on Gherardi went on board of one and returned to New Orleans. Meanwhile he had sent unbeknown to me and gotten the flag. He went up to New Orleans gave the account. We remained at the scene until the explosion which took place about 2 hours after we first boarded her. Here was lost a good prize full of cotton.

There is unfortunately a jealousy existing between the regular and the volunteer Navy. Since our little craft is composed of the latter there was not much made of this matter.

Could the officers have known on board the ram the true conditions of things perhaps the success would have been complete. The *Richmond* whom they supposed would have been at the bend of the river to fight them was there by accident and disabled. Dont think she could have used a gun. Our little craft would have been destroyed I think very easily brave as she was plowing after them. Did look formible as one of the men told me afterward they took us for a boat that had been in the readiness to give them chase. Suppose that we had gotten word that they were on the way and suppose if a vessel did start after them it would have been one fully competent to cope with them. When they found the small force on board and how things existed there was much chagrin among them and some ignored that the *Hollyhock* had anything to do with their capture but because they saw the *Richmond* they turned.

Soon as the explosion took place of the ram we started for New Orleans. Arrived there about sundown. For a short time the old *Hollyhock* was the center of attention her name sung at the theatres and blazoned in the papers. The *Hollyhock* is short of men and more so of officers exception the Engineer Department. It should be remembered she is always, where in commission, under banked fire in town to extinguish fires to run down enemies or

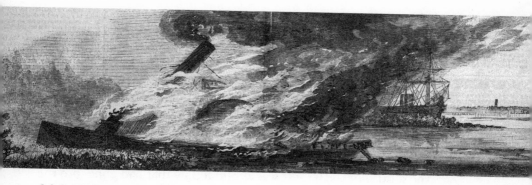

C.S.S. William H. Webb *after being run aground and set afire. (From* Harper's Weekly. *Courtesy of the Enoch Pratt Free Library.)*

do anything that presents [itself to] a dispatch boat [even] to fish up torpedos.

April 25th

On board *USS Hollyhock* Mississippi. Sent down the river to the scene of the wreck of our exploits yesterday. The *Webb* is still burning. We had on board an armed force to see to the escaped crew if the ram had landed them and they brought in Captain Reed and his principal officers who surrendered to our own. Among them was Dr. Addison[41] from Maryland their surgeon. He was hurt in the wrist getting off the ram. I gave him my berth to rest in after giving a little attention to his wound. They will have a giving out of pleasure having been under such stress the past few days. This was a severe effort on their part and from our daring did deserve a better ending.

Later

You will find the Navy registered the *Hollyhock* quotes her 300

41. Twenty-six-year-old Assistant Surgeon J. W. Addison was born in the District of Columbia and a resident of Maryland. *OR:*II:2:155, 157.

tons carrying 3 guns side wheel fast in her day with powerful machines & pumps 30 to 40 crew which was increased at this time by sailors with Gherardi. Ship & crew who had hastily rushed on board make all told 40.

April 26 to end of month spent either in port or on the Mississippi. We would occasionally take a trip down the river. On April 29th on one of these we stopped at the wreck of the *Webb*. Our men got a lot of copper, iron, etc. Also one or two of the solid shot the largest was a solid fellow that had gone into the ram portion of the steamer and embedded itself. We carried it up to Captain Emmons who commanded at New Orleans. He was much pleased.[42]

Undated short time after the chase of the ram

One night went to the theatre in one of their songs heard "but the captain of the *Hollyhock* was the right man in the right place" sung by one of the minstrels. The city papers the next morning gave the *Hollyhock* much credit. One day we again stopped at the wreck of the *Webb*. Our men got a lot of copper brass etc. Some of the men said well if we are not to consider her a prize suppose this might do for awhile. The men got quite a pile of the metal and suppose they soon converted it into a firmer kind. During the balance of the month spent some of my evenings ashore and went twice to the theatre. Sometimes called to see Miss Henrit.[43] During the daytime engaged on the *Hollyhock*. Once during this week we sailed down to the passes of the Mississippi stopping at Pilot Lam [or-Lain].

42. Pasted in the diary here is an article about Gherardi, now an admiral, with his photograph in which he describes fire aboard ship "Fire is my besetting fear. It is the sailor's horror." *(Cosmopolitan,* December 1898.)

43. In an undated entry a short time after the destruction of the *Webb,* Dodson finally named his friend, Miss Molly, as Miss Henrit thus identifying the "H" family. *Hymnal* (Nashville, Tenn.: Abingdon Press, 1993).

4.

U.S.S. BERMUDA

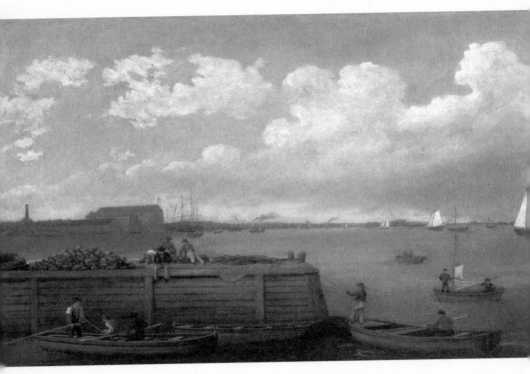

Philadelphia Navy Yard. (Courtesy of the Mariners' Museum, Newport News, Virginia.

New Orleans to Philadelphia
MAY 1, 1865 – JUNE 1, 1865

May 1 to 12

Off New Orleans sailing the Mississippi. This is a beautiful spell of weather we are having. Everything seems so fresh and pure through the country, vegitation so perfect and flowers that we meet with on our different trips up and down the river banks are exceedingly beautiful to look upon. One day in the afternoon when in the city joined in one of the "May day excursions" with some friends and had a pleasant time. The first few days of this month we went down to the mouth of the river. Again everything is unusually quiet on board. Our Chief Engineer is finishing a beautiful propellor cast in brass for some officer who is to have a pleasure yacht. Tis now sometime since I left Maryland and as the war is over I am going up to headquarters to see if I cant go north.

May 13th 1865

Spent the morning on board. Have had a long talk with our officers. They are all Southern men and belonged to New Orleans.[1] They will stay here perhaps until they are mustered out of service. My stay with them has been quite pleasant and ever since duty on board have had things as comfortable and convenient as could be under the circumstances. So in my stay has been many pleasant associations. I told them I was going to headquarters to see if they could let me go off as the war seemed to be over.

---

1. It is surprising that the officers of the *Hollyhock* were all southern men from New Orleans.

Went up to headquarters on Canal Street. Had my discharge from Naval Commandant at New Orleans. He complimented me for my duty and ordered me to the USS *Bermuda* for passage north. So today at 6 PM out of the naval service having been on such duty nearly 15 months.

May 14

This evening found myself civilian and free to move around. Go on board the *Bermuda* and find she will be in port two days or rather will set sail on morning {of} the 16th. Then I went on board the *Hollyhock* got things all ready to leave. Had only to pack up my things as had kept up everything in good order in the Medical Department so as to have nothing to do when the time came for me to leave.

Said good bye to my shipmates. Went on shore had my things placed on board the *Bermuda* then went up town. I had promised Miss M's mother to spend the afternoon and evening with them. As soon as all things ready went there and spent a very pleasant time. I had very pleasant relations with this family during my stay in New Orleans and left quite sorry to leave them.[2]

May 15

Last night slept at the boarding house got things all fixed up.

Met quite a number of friends and most of the morning was passed with a few in the parlor. Had word that the *Bermuda* would perhaps sail a little earlier than was expected. Went down to the wharf and found that she would haul anchor in the stream and the captain wanted all on board at 6 PM so returned up town for a little while longer. Accidentally met Miss M.[3] Went to the boarding house for Mr Bassett who will go to the *Bermuda* with

2. It is also surprising that such a friendship developed with the Henrit family in view of Mr. Henrit's dislike of Yankees.
3. One wonders if this last meeting with Molly Henrit, "Miss H," was

me. So saying Good Bye to all I went on board in time enough for supper on the vessel.

May 16th

They say it was 4 AM this morning when the "anchor came up for home." The first intimation I had was to find myself sprawling on the deck and several persons in the same manner with confusion overhead. When we injured heard we had run into the *USS Richmond*. After a little detention and examination we got clear and steamed down the Mississippi.

When coming on deck later in the day found several old friends and shipmates on board en route for north. Among them McLeary Dr. Smith Dr Shirk also many rebel prisoners from the ram *Webb*.[4] Our destination is Philadelphia. The *Bermuda* is a mail supply vessel coming at stated intervals from the above port and extending her trip to the Rio Grande.

May 17, 1865

Slept well last night and when went on deck found we were nearing Fort Morgan Mobile Bay. We are anchored in the midst of the fleet. Very close to us was the *Ossipee* and *Kickapoo*. On the latter was the late captain of the *Pocahontas*. Surprised to see him. He is in command of this monitor. He has also with him Mr Chandler and could they all come on board and we had a good time.

---

accidental. In spite of his reserved comments about her throughout the journal it appears that Dodson's interest in Molly was more than casual and that it was reciprocated.

4. The officers mentioned on this date have been previously identified. The Dr. Smith is probably E. D. Smith, Acting Assistant Surgeon on the *Arkansas*. Dodson notes without further comment the presence of some of the *Webb*'s prisoners-of-war on the *Bermuda*. The Maryland doctor was not among them. He, Lieutenant Reed, and several others were sent north on the USS *Florida*. OR:I:22:155.

18th off Mobile

Our captain of the *Bermuda* has gone up to see Farragut for special orders.

May 19, 1865

Started quite early this morning for Pensacola. Arriving there we started at 4 PM for our trip for Key West.

20 May 1865

On the Gulf of Mexico steaming along very nicely all going well we all have good appetites and plenty to eat.

21st on the Gulf

Very rough raining quite fast.

22

Came to "Key West." At 11 AM anchored ship. Captain reported at 1 PM. We started sailing out of Key West. Was very good news to us and glad it came so soon.

23

On the Gulf. No land has been seen today we are pushing our way finely for north.

24

On board *USS Bermuda* on Gulf. A beautiful day. Our friends are with each other. We are speaking of the days we spent doing blockade duty at Pass Sabine etc. Dr. Shirk is quite a sight. He went out driving when in the city of New Orleans. Horses ran away and the Dr was badly hurt. He had been fast driving on the shell road at New Orleans.

May 25th

On our way north our dinner today gave poor satisfaction. We gave the cook and steward such a lecture as to cause us to hope there will be no further complaint. Quite a large muster of young men are on board and we are soon acquainted. The wind is quite fresh this evening. Feeling sleepy turn in feeling her steaming along quite finely.

26

They say we are nearly to Cape Henry. The sea rough I know and blowing quite fresh. Still we are driving along at a fearful rate. Came into Hampton Roads as night brings a little moderating. Put to sea again came on to blow very hard had to lay to for hours. I spent this night on deck feeling quite uncomfortable below as the ship rolls so much.

27

On the Atlantic. Very rough sea today. Still we are butting against them and doing our best toward our journey north.

28

Made the Capes of Delaware.

May 29th

Arrived at Philadelphia from which port I had sailed in the *Pocahontas* fifteen months ago. Late in the evening called to see Dr. Mann's family.

May 30th 1865

Spent most of the day in Philadelphia in the afternoon with Miss Ann D———.⁵ Went up to Montgomery County to Professor

5. Apparently Dodson was not too enamored of Molly Henrit, his New

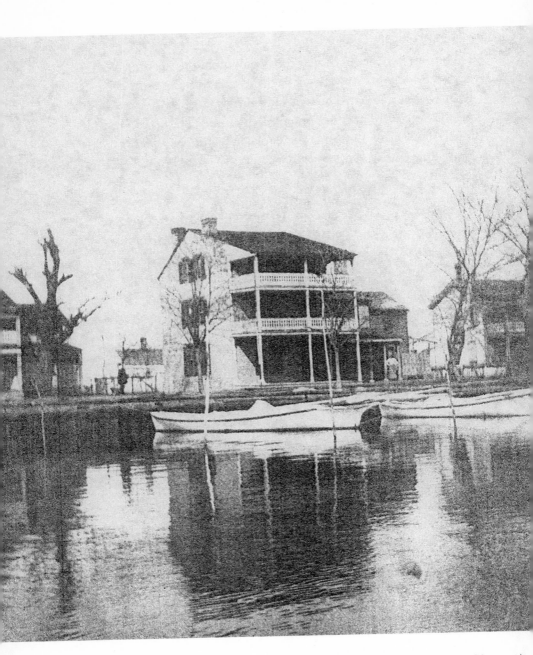

Dodson's house at St. Michaels, circa 1895. (Chesapeake Bay Maritime Museum.)

Sunderland's school. Saw Miss Nellie and Clara. Also took a walk over to see Dr Hahns who lived quite close to the school.

31

Stayed in Philadelphia til 3 PM. Took cars for Baltimore arriving at night. Stopped with Bro Rich and family and tonight expect to mingle in my dreams of home and dear ones I expect to meet tomorrow.

June 1, 1865

At 7 AM went on board steamer *Champion*. Started for home after sailing or steaming as I should have said. [After a] few hours arrived at St. Michaels. Found all home well. I had not given them any notice of my coming so took them by surprise. So here ends my journey that had begun on the same steamer *"Champion"* exactly fifteen months ago.

Here ends the diary but an extensive addenda follows describing the ships on which he served and the symptoms of yellow fever.

Orleans friend, to enjoy again the company of Anne D. Hahn. The other young ladies mentioned may have been Anne's sisters, referred to in the beginning of the journal.

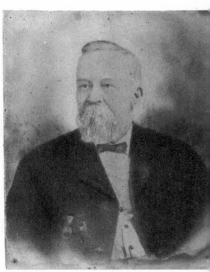

*C. Marion Dodson and his certificate of
membership in the GAR. (Courtesy,
Daniel C. Toomey.)*

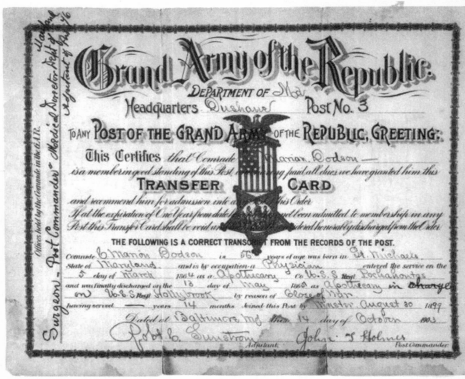

Maryland
JUNE 2, 1865 – NOVEMBER 22, 1929

In the light of his Civil War service it is not surprising that C. Marion Dodson chose in civilian life to become a physician. After the war he attended the old Baltimore Medical College, where he also did post-graduate work in gynecology. He practiced medicine in Baltimore for more than thirty years.

His life-long membership in the Methodist Episcopal Church calls to mind his faithful attendance at religious services aboard ship and his tireless direction of the ship's choir.

Active in veteran affairs, Dr. Dodson belonged to the Maryland Naval Veterans Association until it was dissolved in later years and then joined the Wilson Post, Grand Army of the Republic. He held positions of adjutant, surgeon, post commander, and medical director of the Department of Maryland. When he died at the age of eighty-seven, Union veterans conducted the burial service at Green Mount cemetery in Baltimore.

Dr. Dodson, a vigorous octogenarian, worked on the grounds of his summer place in his home town of St. Michaels, Maryland, on the day of his death. After writing to a son he retired for the night and never awakened. The letter was found by his bedside.[6]

6. Obituary, *Baltimore Sun,* November 24, 1929.

ADDENDA

In the diary, following the chronological account of his naval service, Dodson describes the ships with which he was associated, the mix-up in his records showing him discharged from the wrong ship, and the clinical signs and progress of yellow fever.

US vessels on which I served or was brought in very close relation
From naval register

United States Steamer *Pocahontas*
West Gulf blockading squadron Adm Farragut commanding Captain M. P. Jones, Lieutenant commanding 700 tons 5 guns screw propellor officers and crew near 100 as surgeon's steward one month in charge but not rated.

United States Steamer *Arkansas*
750 tons 6 guns crew 90 to 100 rebel prisoners and refugees 150 As a volunteer assistant in the Medical Dpt on her trip from the Rio Grande to New Orleans with Yellow Fever

US Ship *Fear Not*
over 1000 tons 6 guns at time I was on her guns had not been taken off. She had a crew of about 50 but always receiving convalences from hospitals and fleet to recuperate also a powder supply ship ordered as surgeon's steward in charge to this vessel. She lay off Algiers on the Mississippi.

United States Steamer *Hollyhock*
300 tons 3 guns sidewheel crew variable from 30 to 45 as Surgeon's

Steward in charge B. F. Tarbell Special Pilot commanding Louis Milke Act Masters Mate Ex Officer Alex Wilcox Chief Engineer Frank Boyce 2nd Assistant and a few other assistant engineers

Ida

screw 104 tons 1 gun crew 10 to 20. Not by an official requirement but by an act of my own I used to attend to their crew when she would come into port as she would often tie up alongside of our boat. The two captains being on good terms. In company or at different times we would take dispatches to Mobile Bay. She drew much water and while doing service at Mobile Bay struck a torpedo and sank. I have forgotten how many lost lives but think her Chief Engineer is deceased. I did not attend them as we had returned to New Orleans. Sailing over the same water that she [did] but drawing less water passed over the torpedo with safety. This boat *Ida* took me from the *Arkansas* with my report to Palmer mentioned in the journal.

US *Bermuda*

Ordered to with free passage to Philadelphia as a passenger.

Later

Paymaster T. E. Ryan at New Orleans had charge of several of the vessels accounts and it seems never transferred my name from the *Fear Not* a vessel I was on only two days so my papers at Washington record discharges me from that vessel as class of war and not from the *Hollyhock*.

Yellow Fever

Terrible in its insidious character, in its treachery, in the serpent like manner which it gradually winds its folds around its victims, begiles him by its deceptive wiles, cheats his judgment and senses and them assigns him to grim death. It assumes the guise of the most ordinary disease, a little cold, a slight chill, a headache, a slight fever and after awhile pains in the back.

The misguided victim says "I will not lay by for them." In place of going to bed takes only a mustard bath and a cathartic. He too often keeps up til too late. He has reached the crisis of the disease before he is aware of its existence with the chances thus against him. Then the fever mounts up rapidly and the poison pervades his whole system. He tosses and rolls on his bed and raves in agony. Thus he continues for about thirty six hours. Then the fever breaks gradually it passes off.

Joy and hope begins to dawn upon him and even the doctor may have hope that no return of the fever may occur but if he knows his business may dread even then there may be going on that hemorehagic collection in the patient's stomach which in a short time may be ejected in the form of a dark brown liquid which marks the dissolution that is going on. The fever suddenly returns but now the paroxysm is more brief. Again he is quiet but not so hopeful as before. He is weak prostrate and bloodless but he has no fever his pulse regular sound and healthy and moist skin. A casual observer would think he will get well.

After awhile drops of blood collect about his lips. Blood comes from his gums as a bad sign. Then hiccough which is a sure one. Then follows the ejection of the dark brown liquid generally in large quantity and in 99 cases in a hundred is the signal that the case is hopeless.

Such is about the tropical disease known as "Yellow Fever" raging as a pestulential epidemic and which has so often visited New Orleans and other cities of the South. But the disease may occur, and especially when such a severe epidemic is not in the land, in such forms as to present very remarkable exceptions and differences of symptoms and duration.

While I have seen cases terminate in less than a day after the paroxysm I have seen them linger for several days in a collapsed condition feebleness and irregularity of pulse coldness of extremities intellect clear at times but apathy and tendency to death by asthenia coma and convulsions often occurring at this stage. If death does not take place after these grave symptoms of "black vomit" hemmorhage a recovery is very slow. Yellowness of the surface of the body occurs after the felnle [final?] paroxysm. A yellow conjunctiva with a redness gives the eye a peculiar look.

In my disection at the hospital in New Orleans in November 1864 that died of yellow fever (only to examine the fluids & [viscera]) the times seemed to be found to present the same infiltration of the yellowness color only intensified. Specially the liver is this color mixed ? The stomach is much swollen and showed henmorhage and its results. The kidneys were enlarged the brain and spleen unimpaired. We had to be exceedingly careful in our examination as we would have been no doubt censured by the Chief Surgeon for running such a risk but a few of us who had been attending medical lectures wanted to see a little for ourselves.

One good thing for "Yellow Jack" is that "White Jack" (Frost) in his approach checkmates him and holds his potency in obeyance if it does not destroy him altogether and nothing is so welcome to such as are exposed to that disease than to know a cool frost is coming though it is highly calamitous to patients who are experiencing the disease at that time.

BIBLIOGRAPHY

Baltimore City Directory, 1860

Baltimore American

Baltimore Sun

Boatner, Mark M. III. *The Civil War Dictionary.* 1959. Reprint, New York: Vintage Civil War Library, 1991.

Callahan, Edward W., ed. *List of Officers of the Navy of the United States and of the Marine Corps, from 1775 to 1900, Comprising a Complete Register of All Present and Former Commissioned, Warranted, and Appointed Officers of the United States Navy, and of the Marine Corps, Regular and Volunteer. Compiled from the Official Records of the Navy Department.* 1901. Reprint, New York: Haskell House, 1969.

Department of the Navy. "Navy Historical Center" web site, June 12, 1998, Officers of Navy Yards, Shore Stations and Vessels, 1 January, 1865, West Gulf Blockading Squadron.

Dictionary of American Naval Fighting Ships. 8 vols. Washington: Navy Department. Office of the Chief of Naval Operations, Naval History Division.

Grant, Ulysses Simpson. *Personal Memoirs of U.S. Grant.* 2 vols. New York, 1885–86.

Hamersly, Lewis Randolph, ed. *A Naval Encyclopedia.* Philadelphia, 1881.

Harper's Weekly.

History and Roster of Maryland Volunteers in the War of 1861–1865. 2 vols. Baltimore, 1895.

Holly, David C. *Chesapeake Steamboats: Vanished Fleet.* Centreville, Md.: Tidewater Publishers, 1994.

List of Officers of the U.S.S. *Pocahontas,* April 1, 1864 in List of
   Officers on Vessels, Volume 2, bound manuscripts, Record
   Group 45, National Archives, Washington, D.C.

Lord, Francis A. *Civil War Collector's Encyclopedia.* 5 vols. Harris-
   burg, Pa.: Stackpole Books, 1965–89.

Madaus, M. Michael. *Rebel Flags Afloat.* Flag Research Center,
   1996.

Muster-Roll of Crew of the U.S.S. *Pocahontas,* April 1, 1864,
   manuscript, Record Group 24, National Archives, Washington,
   D.C.

New Orleans Times-Picayune.

*Official Records of the Union and Confederate Navies in the War of the
   Rebellion.* 30 vols. Washington, D.C., 1894.

Tilghman, Oswald. *History of Talbot County Maryland 1661–1861.*
   Compiled principally from the literary relics of the late
   Samuel Alexander Harrison . . . by his son-in-law Oswald
   Tilghman. . . . 2 vols. 1915. Reprint, Baltimore: Williams &
   Wilkins Co., 1967.

Wells, Tom Henderson. *The Slave Ship Wanderer.* Athens, Ga.:
   University of Georgia Press, 1968.

Young, Carlton R. *Companion to the United Methodist Hymnal.*
   Nashville, Tenn.: Abingdon Press, 1993.

INDEX

Abacos, the 30
Addison, Dr. J. W. 127
U.S.S. *Admiral* 39, 50, 61, 62;
   described 61n
Anderson, George 80
U.S.S. *Arizona* 48, 52, 58, 59,
   94, 101; described 59n
U.S.S. *Arkansas* 52, 53, 89, 141;
   yellow fever aboard 73–84; burial
   of yellow fever victims in La.
   59, 80, 81; victim recovers 81–
   83;
U.S.S. *Aroostock* 35; described, 35n

Baltimore Medical College 139
Banks, Gen. Nathaniel P., and Red
   River campaign 37, 38, 38n
Barnes, Augustus, "the knowing one"
   16, 17, 17n, 23, 26, 27, 48, 110,
   112; in charge of Dodson's mess 25
Barton, William 113
Bayou Sara 119
Benson, Charles 6, 11
Benson, George 6, 11
U.S.S. *Bermuda* 20n, 48, 132, 142
Biship, Ed. G. 75n
Blades, Charles 15, 16, 32
blisters, Ceratum Cantharidis, 18n. *See*
   Dodson, C. Marion, medical
   techniques applied by: blisters
Boggs, Archibald G. 21, 21n
Boyce, Frank 101, 142
Boyer, Charles 81
Brazos River 41; and minor cotton

smuggling operations 63, 64
bromated tincture of iron 78, 78n
bronchitis: treated with blisters 18
bronchitis pneumonia 19
Brownell, Edward 12
bumister oxzclate of cennon 78, 78n
Butler, Gen. Benjamin F.: and capture
   of New Orleans 34n

Cadmus, James C. 48
calomel, in treatment of yellow fever
   [n] 76n
Camp Carroll, Baltimore 3, 4, 5
Cape Charles 23
Cape Hatteras 29
Cape Henlopen 22
Carleton, Thomas I. 21, 21n
Carter, Rodney F. 7, 8, 8n 25, 26,
   66, 104, 105, 110, 112, 115
Caswell, E. G. 110
Cate, Lt. David, of U.S.S. *Arkansas*
   75, 75n, 76, 89
U.S.S. *Cayuga* 45; descibed 45n
U.S.S. *Champion* 3, 137
Chandler, Joseph W. 26, 27n, 74,
   133
U.S.S. *Clifton* 52
colocynth, in treatment of yellow fever
   76n
Continental Hotel (Philadelphia) 9
cream of tarter (for treatment of
   smallpox) 112
Crombarger, Perry 24, 24n,
   37, 48, 49

delirium tremens. *See* Dodson, C.
Marion, medical techniques applied
by: delerium tremens, treatment of;
described 23n
diarrhea: treated with castor oil and
opium 95
Dodson, C. Marion *138*; arrives in
Baltimore 3; arrives in Philadelphia 6; arrives in Baltimore
3; arrives in Philadelphia 6; de-
cides to join U.S. Navy 5–7; be-
comes pharmacist on the *Pocahontas*
8, 12; duties aboard USS
Pocahontas 26; messmates aboard
USS *Pocahontas* 25–26; encounters
yellow fever 33; witnesses naval
action 36; describes New Orleans
37; and choir aboard the *Pocahontas*
57, 63, 66, *139*; dissatisfied
with rank and pay 64; transfers to
U.S.S. *Arkansas* 73, 74; treats
yellow fever aboard U.S.S. *Arkansas*
75–84; description of yellow fever
143–44; treats his own fever
94; ashore in New Orleans
90, 97, 107; dissects body of
yellow fever victim 97; meets
Henrit family 96, 99, 106,
108, 115, 128, 128n, 132;
absent without leave in New
Orleans 113–14; U.S.S. *Hollyhock*
92; in pursuit of Confederate ram
William H. Webb 121–25; arrives
back in Philadelphia 135; discharged from USN 132; house in
St. Michaels, Md. *2, 136*; returns
to St. Michaels 137; death of 139
Dodson, C. Marion, medical techniques applied by: acts as dentist
63; blisters 14; in treating
bronchitis 18; boils, treatment of

50, 50n; Fereol's nodes, treatment of
50n; performs minor amputation
63; delerium tremens, described
23n; treats case of diarrhea
95; treats case of high fever
37; treats "Lichen External"
83; treats smallpox in Henrit
family 111–12; treats yellow fever
with compound cathartic 76; uses
lancet 37
Dodson family: brief history 3n
Dodson, Richard S. 3n, 113, 137
Dodson, Robert *3, 4, 5*
Dougherty, John H., aka "Wacuum"
65, 66, 105, 110, 112
Duncan, John W. 33n; contracts
yellow fever 33, 37, 39
Duvell, Barney 28

E., Thomas Tinker 82
Eleuthera, Dodson's impression of 30
Elims, Franklin 91, 109
Emmons, Capt. George F. 113, 122,
128
U.S.S. *Estrella* 47, 48, 110, 116;
described 47n

Farragut, Adm. David G. 34, 72, 84,
119, 134, 141; and capture of
New Orleans 34n
U.S.S. *Fear Not* 90; described by
Dodson 91, 141; attacked by
C.S.S. *William H. Webb* 121
Finlay, Dr. Carlos, and cause of yellow
fever 72
1st Maryland Cavalry 4
U.S.S. *Florida* 120
U.S.S. *Fort Hindman* 119
Fort Jackson (New Orleans) 34n,
119, 120
Fort Morgan 133

U.S.S. *Fort Morgan* 61
Fort Saint Philip (New Orleans) 34n, 119, 120
Franks, William G. 115

Galveston, Tex., capture by Federals, 1862 40n
gamhose, in treatment of yellow fever 76n
U.S.S. *General Price* 119
U.S.S. *Gertrude* 53, 58, 59, 60, 61, 65
Gherardi, Lt. Comdr. Bancroft 122, 123, 124, 125, 125n, 126, 128, 128n
Gorgas, Dr. William 72
Gould, James L. 46, 59
Grand Army of the Republic *139*
Green, Dr. Charles L. 62, 63, 66, 110, 112
Green, Dr. S. S. 58, 58n, 110
green fever. See yellow fever 77

Hahn, Anne D. [n] 6n, 9, 10, 17, 135, 137
Hahn, Frank 20
Hanson, John 90
C.S.S. *Harriet Lane* 41, 59
"Hendon" (musical composition) 58; by Henri Abraham Cesar Malan 57n
"Hole in the Wall." *See* Abacos, the
U.S.S. *Hollyhock,* 91, 93, *103;* case of smallpox aboard 96; Dodson's description of 93, 141; pursuit of Confederate ram *William H. Webb* 120, 121–25
holy stones 45
Hydrargyri unguent (in treatment of smallpox) 112
U.S.S. *Ida* 89, 99, 100, 109, 142;

destroyed by torpedo 113
inanation of the stomach: treatment of 78
U.S.S. *Indianola* 118, 121n

jalap, in treatment of yellow fever 76n
Jones, Meriwether P. 19, 19n, 23, 25, 66, 73, 74, 84, 116, 133, 141; treated for boils 50, 51

Kay, Robert 110
Key West, Fla. 33, 39, 134; Dodson's description of 31
U.S.S. *Kickapoo* 74n, 116, 133

U.S.S. *Lackawanna* 113, 119, 121, 122
U.S.S. *Lafayette* 119
U.S.S. *Lexington* 119

U.S.S. *Manhattan* 119
Mann, Dr. George R. 8, 9, 12, 13, 15, 18, 21, 24, 26, 30, 33, 39, 44, 48, 62, 66; death of and burial at sea 55–56; described 28n; drinks heavily 28, 49; examines Dodson as naval pharmacist 9; illness of 37, 50, 51, 52, 53, 54, 55
Mann, William A. 44n, 46, 52, 55, 57
Maryland Naval Veterans Association *139*
U.S.S. *Massachusetts* 16, 32
McLeary, Thomas 39n, 133
U.S.S. *Mercidita* 21n
Milke, Louis 92, 122, 142
Mississippi River 33, 34
Mobile Bay, Battle of 84n
U.S.S. *Morning Light* 51
U.S.S. *Nathaniel P. Banks:* yellow fever

aboard 82
New Castle, Delaware 22
U.S.S. *New London* 35, 40; described, 35n
New Orleans: 88; capture by Federal troops, 1862 34n; described 37; fire on levee 38; smallpox in 109–10, 111; U.S. Sanitary Commission 100; yellow fever epidemic, 1864 72
Norristown, Pa. 10, 11

U.S.S. *Oneida* 104
U.S.S. *Ossipee* 84, 119, 133
U.S.S. *Ouachita* 119

Palmer, Dr. James C. 85, 89, 90, 142
Palmer, P. N. 91, 113
Pass Calcasieu, La. 35, 35n
Pass Sabine 44
U.S.S. *Pembina* 119
U.S.S. *Penguin* 61; described, 61n
Petrie, Emile 92, 94, 97, 100, 101, 103
Phenix, Dawson 25, 25n
Philadelphia Navy Yard 8, *130;* described 7
Philadelphia, Pa.: Dodson's impressions of 6; welcomes U.S. Volunteers *11*
Philadelphia, Wilmington and Baltimore Railroad 6n
Pinkney, Dr. Ninian 38; described 38n
U.S.S. *Pocahontas* 7, 104, 105, 107, 141; arrives at New Orleans 33, 34; arrives off Galveston 40; blockade duty 36; cases of drunkenness aboard 20; described 7n; described by Dodson 15,

24; desertion among crew 20, 37; dispensary, described 12–13; exchanges fire with Confederate ships 35; former Confederate sailor aboard 14; poor condition of crew 14, 15, 24; fights among crew 39; preparations for sea 12
Port Royal, S.C. 29
U.S.S. *Port Royal* 119, 122n
Porter, Admiral David D., 38n
U.S.S. *Portsmouth* 114
U.S.S. *Powhatan* 14; described 14n
U.S.S. *Princeton* 18

Randall, Abraham 19, 33, 39, 44, 53, 54, 60; description of 33n
Red River 119
Reed, Lt. Charles, CSN 118, 119, *125,* 127, 133
Reed, Walter, and cause of yellow fever 72
U.S.S. *Richmond* 120, *123,* 124, 126, 133
Ryan, J. E. 91, 142

C.S.S. *Sachem* 60n, 61
Sal Rechell (Rochelle salts) 111
U.S.S. *Saratoga* 23, 119
Scully, James 82
Shirk, Dr. Adam 58, 133, 134
Sidney, Charles 110
Smith, E. D. G. 75n, 133
St. Michaels, Md.: Dodson house in *2;* mentioned 3n, 6, 11, 12, 15
"Sunderland College" 10, 18, 137; Dodson's visit to 10

Tarbell, B. F. 109, 141
C.S.S. *Tennessee* 77, 84, 101
Theiler, Max 72
"Thompsonian sweats" 100

INDEX

U.S.S. *Towanda* 13; described [n] 13
Tucker, Anthony 27, 27n
Tucker, Ben 110

U.S.S. *Verona* 81, 83
U.S.S. *Vindicator* 119

Wanderer (ship) 31, 31n
Welles, Gideon 72
West Gulf Blockading Squadron
119, 141
Wilcox, Abraham H. 122, 142

Willey, Thomas 6, 11
C.S.S. *William H. Webb* 117–21, 128;
destruction of 124, *127*
Winters, James F. 110
Wright, A. J., Jr. 28, 28n 112

yellow fever, symptoms and treatment
of 71; aboard U.S.S. *Arkansas* 75–
84; treated with quinine and
spirits 79, 82
Yellow Flag: Dodson's first encounter
with 33